PRAISE FOR *FOODWISE*

"It is often asked whether we should 'eat to live' or 'live to eat.' Gigi Berardi persuades us that we can and should do both, as eating FoodWISE is good for our health, good for the animals and environment in our care, and also profoundly enjoyable. That conclusion is based both on science—remembering that food production is primarily a biological rather than a technical process—and on empathy. As Berardi demonstrates, empathy for other living beings can and should be extended to the animals and people involved in food production round the world, to other workers in the food chain, and to our families and friends sharing our food—through the deeply personal principles, stories, and recipes she shares with us in every page of this life-affirming book."

—MICHAEL APPLEBY, OBE, professor at The Jeanne Marchig International Centre for Animal Welfare Education, University of Edinburgh

"Often the world of food is complex and confusing, with marketing messages that mislead even engaged consumers. *FoodWISE* empowers interested eaters with tools to approach their food in a more thoughtful, sustainable, and healthy way, all the while illuminating some of the pitfalls of our current food system. No fad diets here—just a call back to whole foods and mindful eating."

—MARIE BURCHAM, JD, director of domestic policy at The Cornucopia Institute

"Food scholar Gigi Berardi wades into the troubled waters of advice about what to eat and proposes some truly wise and inspired guidance. *FoodWISE* offers the nuanced, honest answers you'll never get from a diet book, with a possibilist spirit reminiscent of Frances Moore Lappé."

—LIZ CARLISLE, assistant professor of environmental studies at University of California Santa Barbara and author of *Lentil Underground* and *Grain by Grain*

"Gigi Berardi's *FoodWISE* moves beyond inflexible notions of black and white to critically—and unapologetically—examine the gray. By the end of the book, I realized that her seemingly common-sense approach had led me to a profound knowledge about how to be a self-conscious and responsible consumer."

—JASON W. CORNELL, MS, cheesemaker
(affineur)

"For all of us who find ourselves overwhelmed with food choices—'Which apple is most sustainable? Ethical? Affordable? Should I even be eating an apple in April?'—Berardi's *FoodWISE* provides a clear set of unpretentious and practical ideas to guide our eating and cooking. Interspersed with compelling case studies, personal experiences, and sound science, the book reflects an ethic of care for the people and ecological systems that coproduce our food."

—KATE J. DARBY, associate professor of environmental justice and sustainability at Western Washington University

"If you want to be an informed consumer of food, here's your definitive guide. So many answers to so many questions! Berardi gives background to the background—perspective to the perspective—providing a rare, detailed guide to the food world nexus. If you can't figure out what to eat after reading *FoodWISE*, you might as well just stop eating."

—STEVE ETTLINGER, author of *Twinkie, Deconstructed*

"Berardi gently and often humorously guides readers through the intricate threads of the food web from soil to eater, that is, from manure and soil to me and you. Her goal is to share her own expanding pleasure based on a lifetime of the experience: that eating is more rewarding the more we are connected to the source of our food. You and I can tug on threads of the food web if we stop, think, and act based on awareness of mostly invisible people, practices, and relationships that placed an egg or lettuce or a Twinkie before us—especially if we reacquaint ourselves with cooking and gardening. This is a guide, partly about how to choose how we engage with the food system but even more about how to think and act based on knowledge, experience, and good judgment. Although changing direction of the food system requires comprehensive social and policy changes, Berardi helps us make ourselves healthier and the food system more sustainable by aligning our choices toward emerging ways of doing food WISEly."

—HARRIET FRIEDMANN, professor emerita of
sociology at the Munk School of Global Affairs
and Public Policy, University of Toronto

"*FoodWISE* asks us to stop, think, and then act when making food choices. Why? Because every bite we take has impacts on people, place, and planet. To support us approaching our food choices in this way, Gigi Berardi takes us on a journey of self-reflection around our food values and beliefs and how these influence the decisions we make every day in relation to buying, growing, cooking, and eating food. It's also a journey of learning about our food systems, their current complexities and challenges, and what we need to make them more sustainable. Berardi grounds all this, where else but in the kitchen—placing the ability to make a difference easily within reach of the reader. This book gives us practical tools we can use every day to support FoodWISE choices right in our own kitchens."

—C. K. GANGULY (BABLU), executive director at
the Timbaktu Collective, Chennekothapalli village,
Anantapur District, Andhra Pradesh, India, and
board member of IFOAM Organics International

"The dairy industry has changed over the fifty years since I have been in business. The little farms are not efficient, the countryside is filled with empty silos of dairy farms, no longer milking. These small farms are being absorbed by their neighbors—no matter if they are dairy or cash crop farms. The little farms go out of business and their larger neighbors get bigger. The changes in the upper air currents from the tropics and the arctic have led to severe flooding in the central United States—we need to understand that climate is changing. It's made the spring here in New York very wet. I believe there will be a shortage of corn for beef and poultry and hogs, and we may face food shortages and/or severe price increases. Gigi Berardi's *FoodWISE* touches on some environmental concerns but, at its heart, really keeps the farmer in mind. That's what we need right now. Nothing's going to change unless we appreciate farmers and support policies that aid all farmers."

—ED GATES, Seneca Valley Farms, Burdett,
New York

"If you ever find yourself in solitary confinement, or the equivalent, with one book to read, make sure it's *FoodWISE*. Rarely is so much wisdom, common sense, and original thinking elegantly pressed between two covers in a world hungry for food and even hungrier for the full story about the staples of life."

—CHARLES GEISLER, professor emeritus of development sociology at Cornell University

"Why treat nature's food as just another manufactured consumer commodity and agbiz profit center? Gigi Berardi offers a bigger, richer ethic as the centerpiece of a sustainable future."

—JIM HIGHTOWER, former Texas agriculture commissioner, populist author, radio commentator, and editor of *The Hightower Lowdown*

"*FoodWISE* is an incredible body of work—it covers several aspects that I am involved with and that are close to my heart. Berardi takes a critical look at organic farming, climate change, food marketing and fads, vulnerable communities, labor, GMO, and more. Yet, her approach does not paint an apocalyptic picture of the times to come. Without glossing over the hard facts, she successfully creates a multifaceted robust framework that is absolutely logical and critical for our time. At its core, *FoodWISE* is a clarion call asking us to explore the omnipresent agricultural web and aid us toward an experience-based thinking relationship to food."

—MANISHA `MOLLY' KAIRALY, craft and food activist, South India

"More people are becoming aware that what we choose to eat and how it's grown, processed, or cooked has a profound impact on the health of our families and the planet. No other purchase decision we make will have a more profound impact on our present and long-term quality of life—this book really endeavors to connect the dots."

—MARK KASTEL, director of OrganicEye, a project of Beyond Pesticides

"This book is a very accessible and far-ranging primer to help people think about food in a broad context. Gigi Berardi thoughtfully and skillfully explores the myriad ramifications of the decisions we make each day about what to eat, from a flexible whole foods approach to nutrition to important environmental, social, and economic implications. If you want to know more about important issues in food today, and how to make better food decisions, you'll love this book."

"As a sensory scientist, it's exciting to see a food-systems book that takes the sensory experience of food seriously and reminds the reader that the way foods taste are meaningful beyond simple matters of liking and disliking."

"Our small planet faces big troubles—climate chaos, hunger, obscene inequality, and much more. So, it's time to dig deep, tapping the power of hope to fortify our courage. Gigi Berardi's FoodWISE approach—focused on whole farms and foods, trustworthy information, sustainability, deep experience, and empathy—can enable us to take charge: transforming the way we use resources and eat so that we are creating solutions together. That's power!"

"As a traditional dairy farmer in western Washington, I am very encouraged by Berardi's efforts to get *my* voice out there to the non-ag-attached generation coming into society. Although I may see things differently in some of her conclusions—based on science and dirt-under-my-nails experiences—I so appreciate her effort to get students onto *real* farms where *real* people are working hard (and for little reward) to give the populace the safest and cheapest food in modern history. This, while constantly being attacked by either regulators or ill-informed consumers. Getting students to see the effects of broad rules and regulations in regions with many different soils, weather, crops, and practices is imperative. Why? Because the next generation of bureaucrats and regulators need to understand the effects of such rules on the farmer—and at a personal level. Berardi is always respectful and listens to our plights in agriculture."

"*FoodWISE* by Gigi Berardi—ecologist, journalist, shepherdess, and cheesemaker—is an indispensable guide for anyone who wants to make informed choices about what to eat. The author explores food through a wide range of topics: history, agriculture, ecology, sustainability, climate change, food policy, the labor force, and cooking. In her engaging, down-to-earth style, Berardi makes the latest scientific research accessible and the results may surprise you. (Yes, fat is good!) The next time you go to the grocery store, being more FoodWISE, you will follow her mantra to stop, think, then act."

—MOTHER NOELLA MARCELLINO, PhD, Benedictine nun of the Abbey of Regina Laudis and Our Lady of the Rock Monastery is an artisanal cheesemaker and microbiologist, a contributing author to the books *Cheese and Microbes, The Oxford Companion to Cheese,* and *Healthy and Aging,* and she is featured in Michael Pollan's book and Netflix documentary series *Cooked*

"If you've ever pestered the waiter for the origins of that meat on the menu, frowned at the fine print on packaged goods, got dizzy trying to follow the debate on fats and health, or just found yourself falling a bit out of love with eating, *FoodWISE* is the book for you. It's restorative as it is informative, and I love Gigi Berardi's mantra: stop, think, then act."

—MICHAEL MOSS, investigative journalist, Pulitzer Prize awardee, and author of *Salt, Sugar, Fat*

"Looking at problems like climate change, pollution, hunger, and obesity, it becomes obvious that our way of thinking and living is unhealthy. According to Albert Einstein, the solution needs a different way of thinking. WISE and mindful eating is a first step toward a healthy diet from a healthy, fertile soil on a healthy planet. This book is an inspiration and imparts concrete experiences."

—JASMIN PESCHKE, nutrition scientist at the Section for Agriculture at the Goetheanum, Dornach, Switzerland

"Today, on a planet that is devastated by humans, there is no real pleasure without sustainability and awareness. Through her book, Gigi Berardi shows you that a sustainable life is strictly connected to a tasteful existence. Good, clean, fair, and healthy food is the key."

—CARLO PETRINI, founder of the worldwide Slow Food movement and author of *Slow Food Nation* and *Slow Food Revolution*

"What should I eat? With a reasoned approach and careful research, Berardi takes us by the hand and coaches us through this most intimate conundrum. She cuts through the clever speak and ignorance, one theme or fact at a time, to offer a roadmap out of being lost in a million-choice food world. And so, this book equips us to tackle one of the most important decisions we make: what to feed ourselves."

—JOEL SALATIN, Polyface Farms, Swoope, Virginia, and author of *Fields of Farmers, Your Successful Farm Business* and a dozen other books on profitable, small-scale farming

"*FoodWISE* is a passionate, extremely well-informed argument that we should be much more thoughtful about what we eat, for our own good and for the good of our planet. It is full of practical suggestions, including recipes. Reading Gigi Berardi's book will change your approach to shopping, cooking, and eating."

—BARRY SCHWARTZ, professor emeritus of psychology at Swarthmore College; visiting professor at Haas School of Business, University of California, Berkeley; author of *The Paradox of Choice;* and coauthor of *Practical Wisdom*

"*FoodWISE* is a scintillating, readable foray into what it means to eat mindfully, based on thorough scientific research, holistic thinking, and personal experience. Gigi Berardi's wide-ranging exploration of the effects of our food choices on personal health, agricultural sustainability, and climate change is deeply appealing to a biodynamic farmer who has produced most of his own food for more than half a century."

—HENNING SEHMSDORF, PhD, S&S Homestead Farm, Lopez Island, Washington, coauthor of *Toward Sustainable Agricultural Systems in the 21st Century*

"With a refreshing frankness mixed with clear compassion, Berardi navigates the many complexities of food in *FoodWISE*. Starting with the farmers who produce food to the environmental and social considerations of producing and consuming it, to a basic scientific description of food, to ways to participate in a new relationship with it following the FoodWISE principles, nothing is left out of this compelling approach to eating. Using an accessible writing style, Berardi synthesizes a large body of work with her well-referenced narrative that is sure to please and inform both an interested public and the eager scholar alike."

> —RUTH SOFIELD, professor of environmental toxicology and chemistry at Western Washington University

"Berardi does an amazing job breaking down our food ecosystem and explaining what we are actually putting in our bodies. Anyone genuinely interested in eating healthy and being educated needs *FoodWISE*."

> —ETHAN STOWELL, founder and CEO of Ethan Stowell restaurants and author of *Ethan Stowell's New Italian Kitchen*

"As a recent graduate in nutrition and dietetics, I left the US some decades ago to discover Italy and a whole new way of looking at food and eating. At the same time in the US, the "no fat" and "microwave-everything" culture was taking off, and the consequences did not take long to manifest themselves. So many years later, I hope that now *FoodWISE* will help readers to reevaluate what they eat, where their food comes from, how it is produced, and how they prepare it. Certainly, knowing what we are eating and how it is produced is the way to good health, sustainability, and love for the planet."

> —ANN VAUGHAN-MARTINI, professor emerita of food and wine microbiology at Università degli Study, Perugia, Italy

"Gigi Berardi takes her classroom passion for teaching about food and sustainability and transforms it into an accessible message for anyone who loves food! Taking it beyond simply where our food comes *from*, Berardi enlightens all on how food connects us *with* the world around us."

> —GRACE WANG, PhD, academic program director, sustainability at Western Washington University

"*FoodWISE* is the harvest of a lifelong passion for food and farming. It is a cookbook at its best—providing the intellectual, emotional, factual, and scientific ingredients and sharing ways of how to mix them into a coherent whole. *FoodWISE* encourages us to let go of old recipes and considerations so as to create new ones."

—JOHANNES WIRZ, PhD, codirector of the Research Institute at the Goetheanum, Section for Natural Sciences, Dornach, Switzerland, and board member and research director of Mellifera e.V. Biene-Mensch-Natur, Rosenfeld, Germany

"If ever there was a time for people to connect to their food it is now. Food justice is climate justice, and sustainable food production is essential for the healing and regeneration of our planet and ourselves. Berardi helps us get there with this latest treasure—giving us a deeper sense of where our food comes from and how our dietary choices provide a critical connection to this earth."

—JILL MACINTYRE WITT, author of *Climate Justice Field Manual*

FOODWISE

FOODWISE

A Whole Systems Guide to Sustainable and Delicious Food Choices

GIGI BERARDI

North Atlantic Books
Berkeley, California

Published by   Cover art © lena_nikolaeva/Shutterstock.com
North Atlantic Books   Cover design by Jess Morphew
Berkeley, California   Book design by Happenstance Type-O-Rama

Printed in the United States of America

FoodWISE: A Whole Systems Guide to Sustainable and Delicious Food Choices is sponsored and published by the Society for the Study of Native Arts and Sciences (dba North Atlantic Books), an educational nonprofit based in Berkeley, California, that collaborates with partners to develop cross-cultural perspectives, nurture holistic views of art, science, the humanities, and healing, and seed personal and global transformation by publishing work on the relationship of body, spirit, and nature.

MEDICAL DISCLAIMER: The following information is intended for general information purposes only. Individuals should always see their health care provider before administering any suggestions made in this book. Any application of the material set forth in the following pages is at the reader's discretion and is his or her sole responsibility.

North Atlantic Books' publications are available through most bookstores. For further information, visit our website at www.northatlanticbooks.com or call 800-733-3000.

Library of Congress Cataloging-in-Publication Data is available from the publisher upon request.

1 2 3 4 5 6 7 8 9 KPC 25 24 23 22 21 20

North Atlantic Books is committed to the protection of our environment. We partner with FSC-certified printers using soy-based inks and print on recycled paper whenever possible.

For Jim,
Emily, and Ian

CONTENTS

ACKNOWLEDGMENTS

An extraordinary number of family, friends, colleagues, and students have supported me in researching, reflecting upon, and writing this book. These include all the farmers, fishers, food processors, and restaurateurs with whom I have had the privilege to work. This particular project has lasted for six years, and undergone many iterations. Along the way, I have tried to thank all those who contributed to (changing) my thinking. Of course, what looms very large for me are my editors and family (many times, they were one and the same) who have helped enormously in the project.

At North Atlantic Books (NAB), I am ever indebted to Alison Knowles, Acquisitions Manager, for her unwavering support of this project and provision of the resources necessary to complete it. She believed in this project from the first query letter, and has provided invaluable input since. Also, at NAB, I thank Ebonie Ledbetter, Irene Barnard, and Chuck Hutchinson for their editing assistance.

I thank the many who have given feedback and advice along the way. These include but are not limited to Dean Steve Hollenhorst and several of my sixty-plus colleagues in Huxley College of the Environment at Western Washington University (WWU), and, in the final stages of project writing, Johannes Kühl and colleagues in the Natural Science Section of the Goetheanum. I particularly thank Diane Knutson in Bellingham and Torsten Arncken, Mara Born, João Felipe Ginefra Toni, Matthias Rang, Ruth Richter, and Johannes Wirz in Dornach.

I also am grateful for the financial support I received from Vice Provost Gautam Pillay and acting Vice Provost Kathleen Kitto of WWU's Office of Research and Sponsored Programs for funding editing work. Also at WWU, AJ Barse and David Hamiter supplied much-needed technical support (as did

Laron Southcott in Bellingham), and Kathy Thompson helped me prevail over the bureaucracy by providing the necessary documentation to keep me in Switzerland, writing. I am grateful also for the much-needed physical nourishment I received in Dornach, Switzerland, at the time of this writing—from friends at the Anfora Association and from Giovanna Fortuna—which contributed to my appreciation of the beauty, wonder, and enigma that is the Goetheanum.

I am hugely grateful to all my editors—early on Barbara Sjoholm (who helped me refine the acronym title for the book) and Terri Kempton. Terri helped me develop ideas and language I needed throughout the course of the project. Importantly, Terri is the person who suggested I get in touch with North Atlantic Books' Alison Knowles. I am so grateful to Terri for her clever advice, and humor, in forming early ideas into a manuscript.

I thank Andy Bunn, Caterina Dinnella, Robert Lustig, and Stephanie Seneff for their perceptive and helpful review of sections of the text. I caution, though, that any errors or omissions are my responsibility.

I thank my students—fierce food believers, critical thinkers, recipe makers. Many students have read sections of this book, and have not been afraid to give me the feedback I needed. Some of that feedback you can find at https://wp.wwu.edu/gigiberardi/foodwise/student-feedback. The students number in the hundreds and I cannot name them all, but I will give a special shout-out to all those students who made my Ecogastronomy and Food Cultures travel courses possible; what I learned from them, and colleagues on these trips, you can find in these pages. Special thanks to Dan Nessly, who helped coordinate five of those trips, sometimes with Holly Nessly and Kay Sullivan. Dan, a former student and now co-teacher and coauthor, has helped me fine-tune my ideas for the book; I am continually grateful for and inspired by his courage and wisdom.

I have learned much from—and so enjoyed—our potlucks of one hundred-plus students: the food memorable, surprising, heartening, instructive. A special thanks to student tasters (commandeered by Terri Kempton, to whom I am also indebted for taking over my Ecogastronomy teaching while I was on sabbatical): Gloria Baldwin, Andrea Demlow, Lillian Eldridge, Caroline Erdmann, Allie Johnson, Roger Klaaskate, Michelle Matsuzawa, Rachel Montoya, Maya Nash, Miranda Skar, Txell Smith, and Reagan Yonek.

Others, too, exercised kitchen magic: Jim Allaway, Ian Allaway, Heather Graham, Andrews Inglis, Holly Nessly, Dan Nessly, and Teresa Rieland tested many of these recipes and gave vital and much appreciated feedback. Teresa also developed several of the vegan recipes for the book, and Ian and Andrews tested virtually all—a labor of love in such a short time.

I thank other editors, for example, Allison Williams, who joined the team for a time. Each editor helped me in different ways to move beyond complete academic-speak (although, I admit, I'm not completely successful at this) and develop a more accessible writing style. Rose Engelfried and Zander Albertson, however, deserve special mention. Rose—stalwart, insightful— has been a strong editing presence on this entire project. I needed her creative writer's touch, especially for organization, as well as copy editing skills. Zander is a master of teaching and writing, and battled through the editing of the references, as well as the final manuscript proofing—providing countless hours when they were most needed. Daniel Struble expertly edited the Recipes.

I give special gratitude to two of my most diligent editors—Emily Allaway and Ian Allaway. I acknowledge them for how exceptionally skillful (and direct, sincere, and candid) they are in editing what could have been considered, at best, rambling jargon-laden prose. They showed up when I needed assistance most (and best), and I am forever grateful.

Together, these editors have supported me in trying to find the breadth and depth needed to plainly tell the FoodWISE story. They've helped me clarify the material from scientific articles and investigative journalism that I've used to build the narrative. They've supported me in finding less loaded (and more meaningful) words for "healthy," "good" fats, and "bad" science; and in expanding the meaning of others. These include "systems" (the agricultural web) and "guide" (answering questions about Whole, Informed, Sustainable, and Experience-based thinking around eating)—words to clearly state what the book is about (and help us get to our next meal).

Lastly, I thank Jim Allaway. He is both an exceptionally clear writer and an editor extraordinaire. He, more than anyone, has helped me build this material into a cohesive whole. I am eternally grateful to him for his guidance, expertise, and editing—and often with little notice. Gracious and smart, he had a heavy hand in Part 1, and especially the sustainable fish narrative. Moreover, he was present for all the house duties, farm duties, children duties, and sheep duties (of which there were plenty) while I was immersed in my FoodWISE writing world. I look forward to more collaborations with the strongest and most loving writer I know.

INTRODUCTION:
FoodWISE

S ome nights, I sit down at my table and wonder at the journey of the meal in front of me: Here's the fork entering my mouth, there's the kitchen where I prepared all this food. Before that was the store where I selected the ingredients, the trucks that brought the food to the store from the farms. The farms where people planted, watered, tended, and harvested from the soil itself.

Every bite I take connects me to the greater agricultural web of sun, soil, and seed; distributors and sellers; buyers and eaters. That web is a metaphor for the wider network within which we make our food choices. Each of the slender threads is interdependent. Like a spider's web: its high tensile strength allows it to withstand many natural forces, but one broken thread— flooding of a major highway used for food transport, trade policy that supports foreign imports of milk—can make it all collapse. We are *all* part of that web, connected to agriculture, because we eat.

Our agricultural web encompasses the production of human food and livestock feed, and all that we require to grow, process, and distribute it. Certainly, eating means participating in a huge, complex system that ends with us, the consumers. We make choices, we take risks, we allow ourselves to be vulnerable, believing that the food we pick up at the grocery store is going to nourish us. Our very survival depends on our ability to make food choices that will sustain us. For some, our agricultural webs are compact. We want to be as connected as possible to our food and how it's grown or raised. That might mean raising chickens in the front yard, or keeping a goat on an apartment rooftop on San Francisco's Union Street as my college roommate's family did. Whatever we do, though, it's almost impossible to live in a completely isolated way. The larger agricultural web is omnipresent.

On a personal level, we make choices about what to eat, and how much. Dozens of times a day we are faced with the decision of not only what to eat—which food to buy and how to cook it, what to salvage as leftovers and what to toss—but also how much. Agreeing on healthy food choices—what's good for us and for the planet, where to buy our food and how much of it we need—is particularly tough. Indeed, what constitutes "healthy" food is mightily contested, and I try to avoid that descriptor as much as possible in this book—especially in my discussion of fats. Clearly, information about food is everywhere. But a lot of what we read and hear is junk information, conclusions without the research to back them up, or prescriptions for food-related behavior that are just not practical in our real, everyday lives.

As I'm sure you've noticed, results of dietary research change all the time, as does scientific advice—to say nothing of pundits' opinions and food marketing tactics. Had you ever heard of the miracles of açai berry before a few years ago? I hadn't. Around the start of the twentieth century, saturated fat was heralded as one of the most important components of good health. Even early United States Department of Agriculture (USDA) dietary guide-lines touted its vast benefits. Now, saturated fat is widely condemned. But—spoiler alert—it's about to get a serious makeover, as I'll discuss in Part 2.

With all this conflicting information, maybe it's no surprise that many of us are guided as much by our own feelings and ideas about food as by what anybody else tells us. Emotions and information sometimes clash over food—our mood and what we feel like eating versus what we know about what's in particular foods and what's "good for us." How many of us buy that muffin in the coffee shop because it seems just the ticket for what ails us, or have had a bowl of ice cream at bedtime because we feel blue? Mood ups and downs can lead to an awful lot of senseless eating, and it turns out that some foods can reinforce those mood swings. "Blissful" foods loaded with sugar cause the brain to release neurochemicals like dopamine (chemicals that push our pleasure-seeking and possibly even addiction buttons); sero-tonin (the "contentment" neurotransmitter) can easily be in short supply—more about this in Part 2. At the very least, a bad mood can put a certain spin on our food choices.

Personally, to practice mindful eating requires me to reflect on my moods and personal associations with particular foods, examine how emotion, memory, and experience affect my food choices, then enjoy my immediate experience of the moment. Stop—think—then act. For those moments when emotion threatens all good judgment, there is some hard science to point us in reliably wholesome directions—away from processed ingredients and toward whole foods, away from sugar, and away from rampant eating. Of course, there are also times when rational science has little effect—as with disordered eating. Those of us who find ourselves here face a giant set of challenges, where numerous foods or situations trigger overeating or undereating—and I don't aim to give FoodWISE advice for such a challenge. Yet short of these specific disorders, eating too much, eating too little—beyond or falling short of what's needed to meet average physiological and psychological requirements—are behaviors that must be addressed, and I do so in Part 2.

These are the sides, then, in the battle we all fight daily: what we want to eat versus what's good for us, thinking about what we can afford, but also what's available. What we want to eat is shaped by our upbringing and culture, our immediate emotional sensations, what we're used to doing (our food "habits"), and by the blizzard of information and opinions thrown at us by the food industry and commentators—some well-meaning, some self-serving. All of these influences are present in every food decision we make. Friends and peers, anyone we share a meal with, also can shape our choices. Are there foods you "know" you should be eating, like leafy greens, and foods you try to avoid for health or ethical (moral) reasons? Do you have favorite dishes with seemingly magical abilities to heal or comfort you? Our food beliefs can be downright fierce—formed by nurture and the eating environments of our childhood, or adopted through experience and reason in adulthood. These deeply held beliefs and convictions can drive our decisions about food more than actual hunger, facts about nutrition, or economic cost. Questioning my own ideas about food—and the ideas my students share with me—got me to write this book.

As I put down in writing my thoughts about food, I find that often the clearest way to express them is as general concerns that I think many of us share, combined with my own ideas and ways of dealing with them. So I write about concerns for "us," interests "we" have, and about how "I" view them, but also about situations that "you" the reader(s) may find yourself (or yourselves) in and how you might react. Consequently, the writing hops back and forth between first person and second person—that makes sense, because we (that is, I and you) are all in this together. One further note: if you want more information, you will find references in the section titled "Notes" at the back of the book.

In *FoodWISE*, I take a close look at the agricultural web and some of what goes into making informed food choices in it, and I want you to come along on the journey. I can tell you what I've found, but my goal is to help you figure out for yourself how to interpret the things you hear about food. Stop—think—then act; that's my mantra. Don't take anything at face value. Take a moment to breathe and think about what you're learning and how it fits into your life and the things you care about, and *then* act in a way that makes sense—and feels wise—to you.

FIERCE FOOD BELIEFS

I question my food beliefs partly because I know they're fueled by a barrage of messages in media, advertising, grocery displays, and even beautifully scripted menus that all play a huge role in persuading us to buy one food or another in a supermarket or restaurant. Here is some of the conflicting information: Should I avoid fat or double-down with butter slathered on my pork chop? But oil is good, right—especially if it comes from fish? What about vegetarian or vegan diets? Maybe discretionary vegetarianism works best: Do I eat meat when I know the source, but am also fine without it? Do I avoid carbohydrates, or just the sugary, refined kind? It seems like everyone has questions, but not everyone wants to hear advice that contradicts their beliefs.

Before a public address at my university, food writer Michael Pollan asked a group of my students: Why is it that if a cardiologist tells a patient that she's going to need triple bypass surgery, three weeks in the ICU, and a lifetime of heart drugs with a possible risk of early cerebral dysfunction, the patient says, "No problem, I'm in." But if someone tries to advise that same patient to eat green leafy vegetables or stay away from processed foods with their problematic trans fats (we'll talk about this more in Part 2) and more, the response is: "Get out of my face! Mind your own business!" Pollan was talking about nutrition-advice aversion—especially when that advice comes from the medical profession.

Personally, I want to get all the advice I can get—from Carlo Petrini writing about "Slow Food," expounding on the virtues of local foods that soak up their unique geographic identity from soils and water and climate, to TV's Iron Chefs, to USDA policy wonks—because I like food and I like to try different foods. And, I like to challenge my ideas about food. As the advice changes over time, I find my personal food-worldview does as well.

In the early 1990s, I tried to come up with an improved universal theory of food in my book, *Finding Balance*. Instead, I expanded on rather conventional ideas for the time, which seemed like common sense: eat complex carbohydrates such as whole grains and other fibrous plants, and avoid fat. Sugar had not yet been proclaimed our worst nightmare, although groups such as the Center for Science in the Public Interest were valiantly trying to publicize the problem. One of the most effective messages at the time was in the film *Eat, Drink, and Be Wary*, where about 9 teaspoons of sugar were slowly poured into an empty Coca-Cola bottle, showing just how much sugar was in a 12-ounce soda—what looked like a quarter of the whole bottle.

Yet as I was writing about my findings, a Biology department colleague scolded me for getting it wrong. He said I should downplay eating carbs and send a clear message to consume certain fats, reduce others (found in processed foods), and definitely avoid sugars. I didn't *believe* him. While my thinking these days is markedly different—most people now recognize the problems with overloading on sugar—I was doing the best I could with the information I had then. That's how food fads arise and persist: drawing overly broad conclusions from limited information, and not remaining alert to new contradictory or counterintuitive information as it emerges.

I wish I had been wiser then, especially since I do enjoy breaking apart old ideas and considering new ones. Now, rather than seeking a simple food "prescription"—say, the virtues of low-fat, low-calorie diets—I focus on key principles of *how* to think about food. I don't want to push one diet or another, this fad or that; I've learned that any diet that looks like the answer right now may well look ridiculous in ten years' time. Instead, I want to cultivate a practice of critical thinking about food that allows for cultural shifts, an openness to new scientific information, and lets me keep pace with each new food or diet breakthrough. My current thinking on relevant scientific information is presented in Part 2, but clearly this thinking will be influenced by new and additional research. One place to find my current thinking on new research is here: https://wp.wwu.edu/gigiberardi/category/foodwise-resilient-farms-and-nourishing-foods-blog.

Is *this* itself a fad: the questioning of conventional wisdom? Perhaps. But some of us revel in the act of parsing truth from all the contradictions. I believe that carefully looking at information from a range of studies, experiments, and practices, while investigating our own physical and emotional responses, allows us to productively question food beliefs and habits and come to better conclusions for ourselves.

Marketing, current research, family tradition, and beliefs about "good" and "bad" foods determine what we buy, how we cook it, and our overall diet ("diet" in its basic sense: the usual foods we eat—not a particular eating prescription). We need to take control of shaping those beliefs—taking advantage of what science can tell us while acknowledging the complexity of the decision. Maybe if we can figure out the right choices for ourselves, we'll gain the power to change our whole lives just through our food.

As I navigate the new places my plate takes me, I want to follow my own ethical beliefs about the agricultural web, learning from my personal experiences, while taking into account as much science-grounded fact as I can. I'm not sure a principled and experiential approach like this will make me, or any of us, happy and long-lived, but it can at least make us more knowledgeable, satisfied consumers when we recognize—and truly question—our own fierce food beliefs.

EXPERIENCE AND FOODWISE

I am committed to experimenting with food and discovering new tastes. Experimenting, however, is not without its risks. There was the time I ate an unwashed gooseberry in Nairobi and contracted *Ascaris lumbricoides* (it's best not to go into the details of this parasitic worm's life cycle). In Nicaragua the culprit was ice; the setting an eight-hour drive to a remote village during which the only place to hunker down and be sick was beside the road, surrounded by Sandinista soldiers (I won't lie, I was grateful for the cover). In Thailand, during a one-on-one guided trek right to the border of Myanmar and Laos—the Golden Triangle—I ate local vegetables and Mekong shellfish (okay, and some ice—*don't do this*) and got dangerously ill. What saved me was a bottle of Coca-Cola and an elephant I negotiated to rent for longer than the two hours included in the price of the trek. That elephant carried me up slopes so steep I leaned backwards (virtually upside down) and almost vertically parallel to the mountain face. Fun? No. But a good story, and what an adventure! Fortunately, all these stories ended on a happy note—I fully recovered.

My personal misadventures as a confirmed foodie encompass more than illness. There was the lovely cream and fresh-fruit filled cake I insisted on for my July wedding in London—by the time we got to the church it had slumped into a tasty slurry. (A dozen Polish in-laws were not amused, but refreezing the creamy mess resulted in a delicious addition to the traditional menu.) Recently, I unknowingly cooked plain rolled oats as I usually cook rough-cut oats, and ended up with a pot of solid mush. One fall, I tried mixing dry hard cider with a friend's raspberry wine, and got what tasted like weak coffee with too much sugar. Homemade bread with wheat berries I hadn't soaked. Unchilled pie crusts that completely melted in the oven. Yogurt without enough starter to set, which nevertheless became a refreshing drink. So many failed college dishes—just because I didn't pay attention to cooking times, amounts, and was a little too frugal on substitutions that didn't work. (But some did: water, not milk, in my scrambled eggs, was nonetheless tasty.) Overcooked meat—a *lot* of overcooked meat—was especially painful after I had enthusiastically left behind years of vegetarianism.

Does any of this sound familiar? At some level, all of us care about food. We experiment with ingredients and with tastes, we cook and sample and guess. Caring deeply about food need not mean hours in the kitchen and a high grocery bill.

I've made it my personal and professional goal to *experience* food in all its aspects. That experience includes preparing soil beds and working in compost, making cheese, and milling grains. But not everyone has or wants these opportunities. On the professional side, I have taught thousands of students and written many articles and blog entries over thirty years. I've become a book review editor and served on editorial boards for academic journals, as well as started one. I've read hundreds of student assignments and scholarly papers, watched dozens of cooking shows on television, and combed cookbooks and pestered overseas travel hosts for tasty recipes. Has it been a straightforward journey? Never. But my strong relationship with food has kept me ever-curious and ever-cooking. It's gotten my hands in the dirt and my own homegrown vegetables on the table. We don't all have these inclinations or opportunities, so part of my purpose here is to share ways you can consciously experience food with or without the time and money to deeply explore the agricultural web. Why? Because Experience-based thinking is an important part of our FoodWISE guidelines.

FOODWISE GUIDELINES

FoodWISE is really an attitude. Be a little feisty, be a little demanding. Look out for your own welfare. Learn about foods, think about foods, make your own decisions. Everyone can do it. Not all of us can grow a lot of our own food. Not everyone can buy organic vegetables at a local farmers market. But everyone can take more conscious control of what food we put into our bodies—even if that means simply cutting down on constant snacking. Everyone eats; everyone already decides what food to buy and how to prepare it. So what follows are guidelines—admittedly based on my own food journeys—to make thoughtful decisions that inevitably affect not only our personal world (discussed more in Part 2), but also our shared world (discussed more in Part 1) where all our food comes from.

Because I sprinkle these guidelines throughout the book to help you, the reader, in making your FoodWISE food decisions, I have subtitled the book a "Guide." FoodWISE guidelines can be used whatever the venue—whether shopping at box stores, local bodegas, or the farmers market—and whatever the range of food available. But keep in mind that the guidelines are meant to be advisory and helpful—definitely _not_ prescriptive. So much of this book argues against dogma, against simplistic thinking! Think things through yourself, make up your own mind—but please do it thoughtfully, and take advantage of the wealth of reasonable information available.

FoodWISE also is about experiential learning that expands our understanding of the entire food system, from start to finish, from seed to, well, us. By food system, we mean, in food writer Julie Guthman's words: "the entire array of ideas, institutions, and policies that affect how food is produced, distributed, and consumed." That's a pretty big array, including everything from the science behind nutrition to government policies promoting corn biofuels—or what I call threads of the agricultural web. This encompasses all types and scales of producers, and the producing, processing, transporting, storing, buying, selling, preparing, serving, and eating that goes along with food. Then there are waste management activities like composting food scraps or landfilling. The agricultural web is fundamentally an economic system (dependent on and affecting natural ecosystems). And, as Paul Roberts writes in *The End of Food,* there are economic winners and losers. Instability arises. Some players fall by the wayside. Economics and biology affect what food is available. Market Doritos well and suddenly every farmer wants to grow corn. Make a change in the innate pest resistance of a crop plant, and choices in farming will shift. Each of these shifts is a tug on a single thread, yet the whole web moves.

The FoodWISE guidelines acknowledge the greater food system and agricultural web that we are all a part of. FoodWISE centers on some key questions:

Is this food, this system, this meal, or even I myself as the shopper, cook, consumer, thinking in terms of...

Whole? Look for whole grains rather than refined flours; fish and pasture-fed livestock; and dishes that include plenty of vegetables. These foods are generally more satiating than sugary processed foods would be. They also deliver the right amount of fat and nutrients to avoid unwanted and unnecessary body fat, especially abdominal fat (discussed more in Part 2). And is the farm that produced it Whole, too? The "Whole" farm, as I discuss in Part 1, produces crops and livestock, recycles wastes, regenerates resources, and connects to consumers.

Informed? How do we *know* the food we're eating is Whole, and the farm or fisheries that produced it are as well? Being informed is part of a process we all are immersed in—from reading food labels to asking questions at wholesale markets to checking online as to whether or not that store-bought chicken should or should not be washed. One question to ask is how far back we trace our food. I do think there is merit in recognizing all the hidden costs of getting the sirloin steak or rice to our plates. Those hidden costs could include air and water pollution from poorly managed confined (or concentrated) animal feeding operations (or "CAFOs," i.e., with thousands and tens of thousands of animals) and their waste lagoons, or, in the case of rice, long-term health effects of arsenic in rice. Being informed is really about asking questions—and plenty of them, reading labels, and keeping current with research that is thought-provoking and sometimes counterintuitive.

Where did these tomatoes come from, who grew them, how did they get from there to here? What is a genetically modified organism (GMO) and why should I care if I eat one (or a thousand)? What happens when the government funds some dairy farmers and not others? How big is the agricultural web we are a part of, and what does it look like on the ground in our corner of the world?

A FoodWISE attitude values foods that are fresh, local, organic, seasonal, and sustainable—but not necessarily all at the same time. But caution: being food savvy, I sometimes might choose "true blue" (loyal-to-local, but not necessarily organic) over "global green" (mega-farm organic) produce. Doing so helps me be aware of and empathetic to local producers and the challenges they face in providing consistently high-quality produce. Here, I use "quality" to refer to flavor, and to a certain extent, the size, shape, and texture of foods free from contaminants and adulterants.

Sustainable? Are my food choices sustainable for my personal world and my shared food worlds—for consumer pocketbooks and farm expense accounts and maintaining levels of natural resources needed for production, even many generations from now? In our personal worlds, we can't blow our budgets on one week of organic food and think we're going to be fine eating mac and cheese the next week. In our shared world, farms are struggling now, and we need to consider if we really have a sustainable, ecologically minded agriculture when economic viability is uncertain. Economic sustainability for consumer *and* farmer is vital. Changes in state and federal farm policy, which will be discussed later in Parts 1 and 2, can help promote (or undermine) both ecologically minded agriculture and farm/food economics.

Experienced? How involved are we in sourcing our food? To my mind, experience is how we learn best. It is how we learn what we like, how we understand what is good, how we gain our own insights into foods. If experience feels overwhelming or out of reach, start small—talk to people, make a garden in a small space like a burlap sack. It might be just the thing for us non-gardeners.

Experience leads to empathy—the ability to understand and have compassion for other living beings—and empathy results in better decisions about food. Increased awareness of the overall food system helps us to be more understanding of roles within it beyond ours as consumers, and more empathetic to those involved in the day-to-day production of food. Empathy gives us insight into the working lives of fruit pickers, sheep ranchers, artisan cheesemakers, the moms in my twins club, school lunchroom cooks—so we can at least partly understand, both rationally and emotionally, their views and choices. Certainly, when we've done something ourselves—picked tomatoes in the hot sun, milked a cow day after day—we can better understand what that life is like for people who do it full time.

Furthermore, when we have more information (essentially second-hand experience) about some part of the food system, we can make better choices. However, despite extensive knowledge about poor conditions for hired agricultural labor, few federal protections exist—especially true within the federal H-2A program. We need to decide as a society that having cheap fruits and vegetables is not worth the human cost. Investigating where our food comes from helps us assess how much we're willing to contribute in order to ethically consume.

Personal experience helps us make sense of food information and reports of scientific findings. The more we know about a topic, the more we know the questions to ask and the more we can make up our own minds about a particular food. Being critical consumers, aware of our values, feelings, and emotions in food choices, we can be relaxed about food. We can be discriminating but not obsessive, open to new food experiences, and ultimately enjoy the food we produce, purchase, and consume.

MORE ON WHOLE: TO PROCESS OR NOT?

You'll see me write a lot about whole versus processed food throughout this book—me, and the scientists and food writers I draw on. Thinking critically about processed foods is something we need to do as active participants in the agricultural web. We need to carefully consider the connection between the food our bodies need and the food the planet is actually prepared to provide.

Let's start with the food itself. A trip to any grocery—or into many of our kitchens—will reveal a lot of food that obviously didn't just come in from the garden. These foods have been processed, a trend that's taking over more and more of American dining. Whole foods, by contrast, are foods that, when we eat them, are still close to their original state. They have not been processed in ways that change their natural or innate qualities—flour has not been bleached, spices have not been irradiated. Nothing has been taken away and nothing has been added, especially human-made chemicals such as preservatives, growth hormones, or antibiotics.

In the modern agricultural web, both manufacturers and consumers alter foods from their whole state to save time or money or for convenience (canned soup, frozen fruit and vegetables) and sometimes for safety (cooking spinach before it goes bad with slime—a few unpleasant experiences have made me more conscientious). It's hard to argue with safety concerns. The other reasons, though, merit some scrutiny. Take a moment and look at the label on a shaker canister of parmesan cheese. Has cellulose (wood pulp) been added as an anti-clumping agent? Should we care? We're paying for a non-food additive, in exchange for an extra few seconds of our time while making dinner. We *can* trade out those few seconds for a more whole option: dust some additive-free shredded cheese with whole wheat flour or cornmeal, and the cheese will loosen up just fine. We lose a bit of time, but gain a more wholesome, WISEr meal.

Whatever our place in the agricultural web, questions about doing the "right thing" abound. Do I buy the fresh, local produce, even though it may not be certified organic, or go to the chain grocery store and pick up the pre-packaged organic salad greens from several states away? Or take the cheapest option and skip organic and local altogether?

Time is the crux of many FoodWISE debates and practices: whether it be our shopping time, prep and cooking time, time spent in the garden, or in washing the freshly harvested carrots. Less visible is how time shapes the choices of commercial growers. Do farmers preemptively spray their berry fields with costly insecticide—a quick fix—or do they take time to observe, monitor the number of problem insects, and wait to see if spraying is necessary? Or, do they do some of both? Could they absorb the economic loss they might suffer by going organic and not spraying at all?

Becoming FoodWISE means figuring out how to navigate the trade-offs. Stop—think—then act. Depending on money, time, and personal values, everyone's decisions may be different. We all have different experiences to draw on, different resources available, and different values by which we want to live. We embody our own personal FoodWISE systems by examining our beliefs, considering the circumstances and our immediate needs, and developing a practical understanding of why we make the food choices we do. Through these experiences, we become decent cooks, judicious farmers, practical restaurateurs, clever food pantry managers—maybe even observant food writers. And for many of us, this journey is going to start with whole foods.

Whole from Start to Finish

What is "whole" food? Again, it's easy to understand how a fresh carrot from your garden, for example, is whole: You've pulled it from the ground, washed off the soil, and it's ready to go. No post-harvest processing is necessary, and like all the best whole foods, this carrot remains in its natural, non-manufactured state. It has not had any substances, particularly chemical compounds such as preservatives, added to it in processing. If you employ organic practices in your home garden, probably no synthetic chemicals went into growing it, either.

But whole-food eaters don't have to limit themselves to raw carrots straight from the garden. Whole also includes foods that come from animals—any foods that, while they were growing, had few substantive changes made to their natural state. Here, though, things start getting complicated. After all, "few," "substantive," and "natural" are ambiguous terms.

The concept of whole in its strictest form simply can't apply to all foods. Certain foods require some processing to improve their digestibility, or the addition of naturally occurring substances to make them into the food we want to consume. Adding yeast and allowing rising time to create fermented bread, for instance, gives us a less chewy starch that's still crafted mostly from whole foods—and needs only a few ingredients. My favorite *Tassajara Bread Book* recipe (see Part 4 Recipes) has served me well for over thirty years. I might get carried away with ingredients—molasses *and* dried fruit, milk, oats *and* cornmeal *and* wheat berries, nuts, apples. But those ingredients are themselves whole, and a lot fewer than the twenty or more I read on a grocery package (yes, even for breads found in a store's "natural foods" section)—minerals and vitamins, canola and/or soy oil, distilled vinegar, dough conditioners ... right down to components like azodicarbonamide and monocalcium phosphate. Calcium propionate is a mold inhibitor, isn't it? What does "defatted soy flour" mean? Yes, I know that ascorbic acid is a famous water-soluble vitamin, calcium sulfate is a source of calcium, and nonfat dry milk means added protein. But do I *need* the extra protein, and how does it stack up against those whole-food seeds I throw into my homemade bread?

Common foods like bread, beer, and wine require milling and/or fermentation to change the original plant material (here, grain or fruit) to the final food. The enzymes in yeast help carry out the fermentation (although some breads are made with other compounds like baking soda so that the dough rises). Technically, packaged yeast-based foods are processed. But bread yeasts are really enablers of natural processes. Yeasts are natural; in fact they are all around us in the air. It is not difficult to make your own yeast microbial starter, and it is something I do regularly in cheesemaking, but haven't quite achieved in my breadmaking. Any slurry of flour and water will attract wild yeasts, but then again, you might find there are some wild yeasts that aren't going to deliver the desired effect.

Whole also doesn't necessarily mean raw. Cooking is usually a good kind of processing, making some foods, such as meats and legumes, more digestible. Our human digestive enzymes are just right for our omnivore diets but we're not up to chowing down on bones like full-on carnivores. We can digest raw meat, but we get more nutrients once the process of cooking has started the nutrient breakdown for us.

A simple type of food processing is crushing or cutting. Grinding changes the structure of grains, for instance, so that they can be cooked into meal or breads. But if nothing is taken away and nothing is added, the grain is still functionally whole in terms of nutrient value, even though it is no longer physically intact.

Does "whole" mean we only get to eat what's growing in the garden now? I believe in efficiency, and for many of us, efficiency *doesn't* mean planting a carrot seed, watering it daily, and dusting off the dirt months later. It's certainly easier to grab a packaged snack off the supermarket shelf. But what actually goes into making that "food"?

Take Twinkies, an extreme example—as profiled in Steve Ettlinger's sobering, and at times, delightful, *Twinkie, Deconstructed: My Journey to Discover How the Ingredients Found in Processed Foods Are Grown, Mined (Yes, Mined), and Manipulated into What America Eats.* Ettlinger traces the journey Twinkies take to get to our plates as a way of getting us to think about scale in the manufacture of processed foods. Ettlinger describes the eight-mile-long conveyor belts and towering tanks used in Twinkie ingredient transport, tanks so heavily constructed (for transport of chlorine) that some of the steel is 1.5 inches thick. The containers hold mold-fighting sorbic acid; as well as petroleum-derived and naturally derived colors—turmeric from the tuber of a plant grown in Kerala, India, and cochineal derived from the desiccated female cochineal insect collected from dryland plantations of prickly pear cacti. Then there's vitamins—and Ettlinger describes how most of the world's niacin comes from Visp, Switzerland, from a liquid petroleum gas/naphtha and petrochemical plant—more big tubes, towers, giant tanks, catwalks, and ladders. More important than the look of such (big) scale are the resources that are corralled to produce the sweet treat. Mountains are literally moved to mine all these chemicals. So, what's in your Twinkie? A lot of resources, a lot of labor—and very little whole food. This may be an extreme example, but the lists of ingredients added to processed foods are impressively large.

If we want to keep our mountains intact and limit our petroleum consumption, does that mean we have to go non-processed all the way? Not at all. There are alternatives to mined powders and hefty amounts of distillates that are used to preserve food at home but also commercially. Throughout time, people have preserved foods by pickling, salting, sugaring, and smoking. Sulfur dioxide has been added to wine to stop fermentation and solve the problems of exploding bottles and microbial growth (something I've learned about the hard way), and copper sulfate is used to control mold on growing plants. I don't particularly care for either—there are other ways to preserve and protect—but I still call sulfured grapes (again, I'm not a big fan of exploding bottles of red wine) and raisins "whole."

That leg of mutton stashed under the thatched roof above the smoky peat fireplace of an old Scottish cottage would have provided whole and wholesome (if tough) food many weeks after slaughter. For centuries, people in Italy produced salamis and sausage using only natural preservatives such as salt, pepper, and spices. That was whole food. But today's common commercial practice of preserving meat with additives such as nitrites and other chemical compounds yields a product that can only be considered adulterated. Nitrites, for example, are used partly to enhance the red color of meat products and make them look more appealing. They also inhibit growth of bacteria. Nitrites, however, are not a remedy for poor plant processing hygiene. Turn-of-the-century food safety laws, including the Pure Food and Drug Act and the Federal Meat Inspection Act, both of 1906, were meant to prevent adulteration and mislabeling of foods and encourage good hygiene and sanitation in plants.

Chilling, and certainly freezing, fresh meat or cheese slows bacteria growth and enzyme breakdown. It's a form of processing that allows food to be transported across long distances, kept reasonably fresh over time, and made available to consumers worldwide who don't have daily access to fresh meat or carrots growing in their gardens year-round. Foods handled in these ways certainly can still qualify as whole, even though some aspects of their makeup have been altered. By contrast, pasteurizing milk to kill pathogenic and spoilage microorganisms renders it less Whole. There are several methods of pasteurizing; vat pasteurizing at a lower temperature for a longer time preserves more physical/chemical properties of the milk—the milk is, for example, more suitable for cheese making.

The key to maintaining the wholeness is to not add foreign chemicals to enhance flavor, appearance, or shelf life. I am not interested in ultrapasteurized milk that can last for months, even if it is organic. Yes, it works economically—ultra-pasteurizing enables long-distance transport and long shelf life, which is necessary for some consumers in remote areas. And yes, if such treatment results in a lower price for "organic" milk—albeit from the largest-scale producers that reap the greatest returns—then, sure, that low price is appealing to many of us. But does "cheap" need to be the default?

I am fortunate to live in a region with options, so I'd rather buy something fresher, not ultra-pasteurized, something that's the product of probably a lot more pasture than used by big corporate "organic" farms. More expensive? Yes. And so I just drink less of it. With all the nutrients that sunlight, real grass, and grazing cows have packed into that milk (in particular, desirable fatty acids), I have concluded that I can drink less and still get the same healthy results—which somewhat mitigates the additional cost. For me, the choice is a combined question of values and economics, and reflects my FoodWISE approach.

The trick here is to stop—think—then act; consider all the factors in play and make your decision from there. For me, local, pasture-raised dairy is a priority, due to the favorable fatty-acid profile and the ordinary animal behavior of cows grazing. But I don't just drink my milk straight—I'm a cheesemaker, after all. And I still consider fermented foods such as yogurt, cheese, and sauerkraut to be whole foods. Natural processes of fermentation are everywhere. Milk wants to be cheese and sour cream: it starts to sour soon after it exits the animal unless properly refrigerated and handled. Cultures aid the transformation.

That is the origin story of cheese: probably discovered millennia ago by some traveler in the Middle East who set off for the day carrying milk in the handy container of a calf or sheep stomach, and found at the end of her journey that it had turned into something quite different, and quite tasty—curdled into the beginning of cheese by the rennet coagulant naturally in the animal's stomach. No mountains mined, no massive transport vehicles needed to make this delicious food—"making" cheese this way just means helping milk do its thing. That's the kind of processing I can get behind as a FoodWISE consumer. And as a cheesemaker I do—in the springtime, almost every day.

Whole While Growing

We've been thinking about what happens to a food item—be it grain, nut, fruit, vegetable, chicken, or egg—after it is harvested. But the same Food-WISE principles apply to the plant or animal *while* it is growing: don't change its nature, and don't add chemicals to enhance flavor or growth. In some cases, this is as simple as not spraying any herbicides in your backyard gardens or on your cornfields. But this measure of wholeness applies to animal agriculture, too.

Wholeness values connections between farmers and their flocks and herds. Connection means farmers are linked (physically, onsite) to their animals. They can determine firsthand which individuals are ready for slaughter and market and which are vulnerable to disease and digestive disorders.

Large, confined animal operations, referred to as CAFOs, can be classified (for regulatory purposes) according to the number of confined animals. Typically, in large operations, the flocks or herds may have little opportunity to express their "animalness" (normal animal behavior): their ability to recognize individuals in the flock or herd or to forage (in the case of chickens) widely for feed. Even with the organic label, in some situations, the animals may have only minimal access to the outdoors. "Pastured"-labeled chickens, for which you know something about the scale of operation (this is key), and the extent to which animals have free range to outdoor fields and grass, might be the best choice.

Experience huge chicken operations and you may be inspired to start your own backyard egg-laying project. I certainly was. Does this mean we need a chicken in every yard? Well, not exactly. But enormous chicken operations are rarely the only alternative. Smaller-scale works, and within thirty minutes of where I live, two growers keep 250–600 chickens at a time. The chickens are out in the field, where their "chicken tractors" (movable fenced-in protective units—with nesting boxes if the hens are laying) are large enough to allow for some natural behavior. This promotes good health and physical comfort for the chickens. Agricultural populist writer-farmer Joel Salatin calls this "integrity farming." With animal products, what we consider whole is sometimes partly a question of our attitudes toward non-human animals.

FoodWISE is choosing to consciously consider what we consume, keeping personal budget, values, and tastes in mind. But what is the right number of chickens to be raising? If 10,000 is too many, how do we know 600 is not? We don't. This brings us back to the FoodWISE approach—Experience it for yourself. What's *your* observation? If you don't happen to have local chicken farms in your area, take a look on the internet. Just type "chicken farm tour" + your geographic area in your web browser.

Strict application of FoodWISE guidelines rules out food from plants or animals that are genetically modified organisms (GMO) or genetically engineered (GE). For one, we don't know what unintended effects might follow from altering the genes. Is animal consumption of GE corn and soy—genetically modified to make it resistant to the herbicide glyphosate (as in the popular product Roundup that is used to kill competing weeds in the fields)—any different from that of non-GE corn and soy? Apart from that uncertainty, there is increasing concern about contamination of nearby crops by airborne pollen from those GE plants. The effects of glyphosate remain vigorously contested. As I mention later in the Notes, some researchers deliver a strong verdict on certain aspects of this.

Using certain insecticides, herbicides, and fungicides to disrupt inherent biological cycles or using irradiation for preservation puts food over the line, taking it from whole to contaminated. But hold on! Does that mean *no* chemicals? No. It just means we have to be careful about the ones we choose.

We do know that the widespread use of antibiotics and growth hormones for livestock has led to the development of antibiotic-resistant pathogens, meaning it's getting harder all the time to kill harmful bacteria. Environmental damage from widespread chemical use also continues. It's no longer DDT residue threatening the reproduction of bald eagles—thank you, environmental pioneer Rachel Carson (aided by Marjorie Spock). Now it seems to be amphibians around the world threatened by other endocrine-system hormone disruptors, and a host of other emerging crises.

More directly related to our own food-shopping decisions is the worrisome place of strawberries, spinach, nectarines, and apples at the top of the Environmental Working Group's "Shopper's Guide" to the "Dirty Dozen" list of fruits and vegetables contaminated with pesticides. Certainly, washing apples in baking soda and water removes some chemicals, but other residue may penetrate the flesh or seed. And some produce is so difficult to wash that we are often tempted to skip this step altogether.

Does this mean that we can't add anything to our farms to help plants grow? Does whole-food farming mean leaving plants to fend for themselves? Not at all. Plants grown using plant or animal composts still qualify as whole foods. Adding nutrients through compost isn't adulteration, but rather natural recycling, using only compounds that would occur in a typical, whole-farm ecosystem. Soils that food crops are grown in often include some decomposing plant matter, and that soil is being processed by animals like earthworms and a host of other organisms. As for added animal manure: bring it on (and hopefully in reasonably dry weather) and preferably in "agronomic" (carefully planned) amounts, suitable for what the plant needs. Decomposition of animal manure is a major pathway for recycling nutrients in natural ecosystems—and once again, adding manure just means adding more of what these plants would absorb if left to their own devices.

I'm not saying that farming necessarily should look like it did 200 years ago. I used to have a hard enough time keeping the cow/goat/sheep poop out of my milk pail in the morning—I can't imagine what to do with the mule manure in threshed grain in a turn-of-the-century millhouse. However, in terms of soil fertility management and healthy food, a less artificial, more on-farm, biology-based system seems key to both short- and long-term sustainability.

Edible yeasts plus edible whole-grain flour make whole-food bread. Yeast plus processed flour plus BHT plus caramel coloring plus hydrogenated vegetable oil plus vital wheat gluten plus unspecified "enzymes" do not. By supporting whole foods, we can work within the food system to strengthen those particular production threads in the web. This also is important in our personal worlds, which we will discuss more in Part 2. There's nothing like the personal experience of having dived wholeheartedly into several diets, heavy on processed and low on whole foods, only to be serially disappointed, to make us skeptical.

A WINDOW INTO MY BELIEFS

I like to eat real food—I like to know where it came from, I like to think about the county or farm or farmer of origin when I'm eating the food. I enjoy growing my vegetables and raising lamb. I also am quite clear on why not all families still produce much, or even any, of their food. It is time-consuming, difficult, exhausting, and risky. Shopping and cooking also take time and energy. I get the draw of convenience. I like inexpensive as much as the next person does. And I know we wouldn't get either convenience or cheapness if we were all in our kitchens cooking everything that went into our mouths.

My father was part of a large Italian family. My mother was born in Arkansas and grew up in Oklahoma. As a teen in 1922, she moved to California on her own. From grits to *lasagna suprema,* my mother was a great cook. She lost her Ozark accent and, literally escaping the Dust Bowl, started a new life in Hollywood (where I was born). She no longer raised crops or loosened soil—but she did marry an Italian romantic and nurtured my sister and me with arguably the world's best food. She exposed us to a huge variety of tastes and we never went hungry—unlike herself and her brother and sisters.

On any one day, my mother might be making two separate suppers so both my sister and I could get whatever food we craved. Then my father would come home and cook some Italian dish like roasted fennel, pasta and beans *(pasta e fagioli),* or vermicelli with anchovies. With all these parallel meals, the possibilities for sampling and experimenting never ended.

The cooking captivated me, as did the shopping. Going to the small market as a little girl was a great adventure—but nothing compared to going to the new Vons supermarket in Burbank, California, with its colorful aisles and huge delis. Spectacular though it was in my child's mind, big stores like this cut out our weekly visits to what we called "the Italian store." No more trips to retrieve fresh, raw milk at the Alta Dena Dairy either, or daily orders left for the back-door milkman. As a child, I have to admit I welcomed the creep of convenience foods into our home. Pop-Tarts and processed breakfast cereal—vivid memories.

I know a lot more about food now, and that's due, in part, to my life experiences in other places I also have lived. Besides southern California, these include upstate New York, central Maryland and the greater Baltimore area, rural western Pennsylvania, and Southcentral Alaska. In each locale, I have found FoodWISE food and farms. I need to make this clear because a lot of my references here are to the bountiful Pacific Northwest—but I have developed my FoodWISE thinking by living elsewhere.

Today, I still decide what to eat based on what tastes good. I enjoy the fresh fava beans from my friend's garden on Orcas Island, the crispy sprouted almonds I prepare myself, my partner's venison, the dandelion wine I make in memory of Ray Bradbury's fantasy novel on whatever day of summer I choose for the harvest. These foods taste good to me. They also involve a little bit of cooking, handling, and experimenting. They make meals not just a task in the day but part of that day's experience, allowing me to participate fully in the agricultural web—not unlike my mother's weekly visits to local farmers and grocers when I was a child.

I think a lot about my mother when I'm in the kitchen, and whenever I'm exploring the larger world of food. I'm reminded of her when I read works by people like food writer and gastronome extraordinaire M. F. K. Fisher, with whom I share my no-nonsense approach to cooking. I love this quote from Fisher's *How to Cook a Wolf,* about the value and dignifying nature of cooking, which allows us "to nourish ourselves with all possible skill, delicacy, and ever increasing enjoyment. And with our gastronomical growth will come, inevitably, knowledge and perception of a hundred other things, but mainly of ourselves."

I, too, believe the same.

I believe whole, unprocessed food is nourishing.

I believe in making my own food when possible.

I believe that the more connected I am to the source of my food, the more rewarding my experience of eating can be.

I believe you can find that connection, too.

BEING FOODWISE IN THE KITCHEN

Lofty philosophies only get us so far if we don't put them into practice, so being FoodWISE in the kitchen means being realistic about what you can and can't do. Stop—think—then act. We won't all make the same choices—we don't all live the same lives! What we can do is foster the FoodWISE attitude: a little feisty and a lot informed.

That doesn't mean that low price and convenience don't matter. They do. Inexpensive organic is welcome, yes? Yet, our grandparents (mine at least, from rustic Italy) would be horrified at the idea of shopping for plastic-wrapped tomatoes that still aren't ripe when you bring them home, or valuing "organic" produce from massive farms.

Then there's the phenomenon of Trader Joe's (the grocery store company). While I don't mean to knock lovers of "Two-Buck Chuck" (wine), I have to point out that Trader Joe's—its produce and products consumed by many—is too conveniently just around the corner for many. The chain's message can be insidious: don't cook tonight, we have *so much* prepackaged, ready-made (and delicious) food. Throw your dinner parties, feed your family "healthy" snacks and cheap, chic wine.

Further, we've seen a flood of "greenwashing"—labels touting many "healthy" or "environmentally sustainable" things when it's mostly just deceptive spin. Sometimes it's difficult to distinguish between what's greenwashing and what's real. Being FoodWISE doesn't mean knowing every environmental fact about food, but rather being curious at least about how food is produced and prepared—even if this means merely knowing what type of animal produces your veal cutlet.

If you are deeply and passionately involved in eating, perhaps with family and friends, then knowing how to cook and where your food comes from is part of being informed. As you shop more (and more knowledgeably), you'll learn about what grows near you and when, how to prepare different fresh produce and meat products, which items must be used immediately, and which last a few days. You may start seeing things a little differently. For example, you may realize how strange it is to expect a ripe avocado or sweet orange out of season. FoodWISE shopping goes hand in hand with our lessons about farming. Losing that intuitive connection with the seasons and the availability of certain items is the price we've paid for things like convenience and long shelf life.

Cooking FoodWISE isn't whipping up a perfect soufflé or staging Instagram-worthy plates. It's learning to put together some tasty whole food dishes, even if with just a few, simple ingredients. It's finding sources of local and fresh foods, and becoming familiar with what's available in what seasons. It's experimenting with a few new foods or ways of cooking, even if just a little bit. It's connecting with your friends to learn about other places to find ingredients, or other ways of preparing foods you're familiar with, or new dishes altogether.

How we value time is also critical to the FoodWISE debate and practice—in the kitchen, on the farm, at the store. Do farmers buy chemical pesticides so they can spend their energy and labor elsewhere? With our own food choices, do we invest in shopping and carefully preparing by hand an intricate menu, or just heat up something in the microwave?

These conflicts and choices are part of our every day, and I cannot advocate strongly enough that we start reinvesting more time in food preparation and enjoyment. How else to develop kitchen savvy? You get more practical experience and wisdom by boiling some water, even to make mac and cheese from a box, than you do sticking a bag of premade food into the microwave.

That's right—I am advocating a package of macaroni and some boiling water as a substantive cooking experience, particularly if you experiment (add some pepper?). Even this, to me, is cooking. Is it Whole? Just take a look at the ingredients on the box: not exactly. So, ixnay on the "W" in WISE, but bring on the "E" for Experience—you're cooking! And maybe, after reading this book, you will have the "I" for Informed and the "S" for Sustainability, which might make you rethink stocking up on the highly processed version of that cheesy mac.

Becoming FoodWISE means becoming conscious of the ways our decisions shape both our shared and personal worlds. In Part 1, we'll look closely at how food is produced in our shared world. I want to start big, looking at that agricultural web and how our food choices can relate to it. We'll zoom in on food in our individual lives in Part 2: what diet culture means, what science does (and doesn't) say, and how the beliefs we've grown up with shape our decisions. Finally in Part 3, we'll stop—think—then act, using FoodWISE guidelines. In Part 4, I share recipes. How do we put all this into practice and become conscientious, responsible eaters—and good cooks—in this world that is so full of delicious food?

PART 1

Our Shared World of Food and Farming: Choosing Whole and Sustainable, from the Ground Up

The WISE approach to food choices is something we put into action many times a day: growing, buying, cooking, eating. We'll do it again tomorrow, and the day after tomorrow. And our children will do it daily in years to come, and their children after that.

So an agricultural web that allows us to make good food choices has to continue to exist into the future, it has to persist. The entire agricultural web of producers, transporters, processors, sellers, and consumers has to be sustainable.

For today's agricultural web to be sustainable into the indefinite future, a lot of things have to go well. Land has to be available and the soil, water, and air have to be right for food production. Financial incentives have to be adequate for farmers (and fishers) to produce whole food in a sustainable way. Incentives also need to be in place for processors and wholesale and retail suppliers to provide food sustainably. And every part of the system needs to be resilient to be able to adapt to changes as they come along. Finally, consumers need to have the financial ability, the opportunity, and the knowledge to buy, cook, and eat what they consider to be good food.

Because this is an integrated web, feedback from every step up the chain provides incentives (or discouragement) to every preceding step, and that feedback helps decide what happens there. Processors make and offer for sale the kinds of foods that consumer demand tells them to. Farmers grow more of the crops that make them more profit. In addition, many other influences exert constraints or incentives in the web: land use (or fishing) restrictions; competing uses that offer higher land prices than farming, like high-end residential housing; crop subsidies and other government support programs that favor particular crops or particular kinds of farms (mainly large ones); and a big one: external forces—global markets and prices, political crises, and other issues affecting food production from around the world.

The big outside force we face now is the world's warming climate, resulting from decades of human production of more greenhouse gases than natural systems can recycle. A warming climate can cause even more changes to the world's agricultural web—and likely your own local food system—than we can imagine. But we can try to foster sustainability and resilience so as to cope with coming changes.

Part 1 is intended to give some insights into how the vast and complicated food system, previously discussed in the Introduction, works and how it got to where it is, highlighting which particular aspects are or are not sustainable. A key way to achieve sustainability is to be resilient, and that includes changes in how governments can support the food system.

WHAT IS SUSTAINABILITY?

Something is sustainable if it can keep going, maybe indefinitely. When applied to the food system and particularly farming, "sustainable" refers to a system of production that maintains or enhances food-producing resources—mainly soil and water—while maintaining yields. Soil is likely to be suitable for sustainable farming when it remains fertile, high in major nutrients like nitrogen, potassium, and phosphorus but also calcium and magnesium; and contains abundant microbes to produce and recycle organic matter. Maintaining an intact and porous soil structure even when exposed to wind and water—the big movers of soil—also is important. Organic matter, with its large capacity to hold nutrients and water, contributes to all these elements that make soils good for sustainability.

Ideas that current farming practices should enhance the natural resources—particularly soil—needed for future generations have been around a long time. In the early twentieth century, ideas of integrated production—with the various parts of a farm all working together and supporting each other—gained momentum in Europe following the influential Agriculture Lectures of Rudolf Steiner in 1924, and eventually grew into the biodynamic movement. During the Dust Bowl years (1930s) in the United States, the Soil Conservation Service was created in an effort to inventory, protect, and rehabilitate the nation's soil resources. "Organic" agriculture surfaced in farming literature of the 1950s, bolstered by Robert Rodale's work in regenerative agriculture. His ideas were developed to counter the rapid industrialization of agriculture following World War II by emphasizing the renewal of natural systems without the use of synthetic chemical inputs that might compromise biological processes. About the same time, in the 1940s, Masanobu Fukuoka, a Japanese plant pathologist, philosopher, farmer, and writer, was developing his ideas of farming without cultivation and chemicals, rejecting typical techniques for, say, rice production that involved flooding of fields; and instead developing a more "natural" form of farming. His 1975 landmark work, *The One-Straw Revolution,* greatly increased interest in sustainable farming.

Since then, dozens of writers and farmer-authors have discussed the need for sustainability in farming, arguing against short-term gains based on unsustainable political and economic practices. I've spent a lot of time in my professional life looking into questions involving sustainability and resilience. I'll talk about some of these projects and what I've learned from them as we get deeper into this. For me, resilience is the ability of a community or system to withstand threats. Resilient systems are sustainable, but also show adaptive capacities to become even more resilient once a threat has occurred.

One of the biggest threats to agricultural webs is climate change. Current patterns of food production will change around the world as seasonal temperatures and rainfall change, and increasingly food may be hauled from farther away. The greenhouse gases that agriculture produces are a big concern. Food production is one of the top sources of greenhouse gases such as carbon dioxide, methane, and nitrous oxide that contribute to the increase in global temperatures currently threatening our planet. It is easy to see some of the reasons for why this is so: Larger livestock feedlots concentrating even greater amounts of methane emissions and transporting food (long-distance transport of foods but also short-distance transport from supermarkets to your home refrigerators) produces carbon emissions.

United States agriculture has been a great success story in recent decades in terms of increased yields. Problems come from how the food is produced in the first place and who gets it—and whether these levels of production can continue.

IS GOING BACK TO ORGANIC FARMING AN ANSWER?

Since a lot of the difficulties in achieving food sustainability result from depletion of natural resources and damaging impacts on the environment from a more industrialized agriculture, organic farming has often been assumed to be a big part of the solution. Organic farming, after all, centers on using natural processes for fertilizing and maintaining the structure of soil, and avoiding use of unnatural substances like synthetic pesticides.

The demand from consumers for chemical-free food has boomed in recent decades. Organic farming has grown and evolved in response, but still has a ways to go. By 2016, the total acreage of certified organic farms in the United States had increased to five million acres. As big as that number sounds, it's only about 1% of all arable (farmable) land. US farms and ranches accounted for $7.6 billion in certified organic commodities (think poultry, milk, and eggs, but also lettuce, tomatoes, and corn). Apparently, almost 40% of US adults say that "most" or "some" of what they eat is organic.

But let's look more closely at the assumptions consumers have about the sustainability of organic farming. It may, in fact, be part of the solution but the situation is more complicated than it seems at first glance.

We define "organic," in large part, by what it is not. Organic farming, by and large, does *not* use synthetic chemical insecticides, herbicides, or other pesticides. It does *not* involve the use of irradiation (this relates particularly to organic food processing) or genetic engineering. The purpose of all this, in the words of the USDA, is to "integrate cultural, biological, and mechanical practices that foster cycling of resources, promote ecological balance, and conserve biodiversity."

Any farmer can follow these practices. But to legally sell food products in the United States that are labeled "organic," a farmer must pay to have his or her operation formally *certified* by an official body such as the USDA or state departments of agriculture, or nonprofit organizations such as California Certified Organic Farmers. The requirements for certification typically include that at least 95% of the food product be produced organically, as described earlier (which of course means up to 5% may not be).

The upshot is that there's a difference between farming organically and being formally certified by the USDA as "organic." Some commercial farmers who think it's not worth the trouble and expense don't bother with certification but still use organic practices. That's why all sorts of similar-sounding descriptions appear on food labels, particularly in small markets: "Grown Naturally," "Raised Without Antibiotics or Hormones," "Pesticide Free." In fact, a handful of independent certifying programs aims to provide simpler and cheaper certification for *essentially* organic production. See, for example, Certified Naturally Grown's program at www.cngfarming.org. Just because a food for sale doesn't have USDA organic certification doesn't mean it hasn't been produced using standard organic practices.

Organic certification continues to be the subject of controversy. Among its present weaknesses, my favorite irony is that wild salmon, born in a mountain stream and maturing somewhere out in the Pacific Ocean, cannot be labeled "organic" because nobody—the fishers who caught them, the market selling them—can prove that they were raised without pesticides, chemical additives, or in accordance with the other criteria.

But here's the main thing about "organic" certification from a FoodWISE perspective: "Organic" does not necessarily build farm communities or promote integrated, reduced-external-input farming. Many large organic farms actually look an awful lot like their nonorganic mega-scale counterparts. (In later sections, I talk about small-scale, integrated farms that often are tied into their communities, in contrast to very large-scale or mega-farms.) So, some growers reject certified organic production, choosing to be "beyond organic" by doing more than is required.

Remember the purpose to conserve biodiversity that was included in the USDA "organic" definition? Well, it turns out that doesn't necessarily mean a multispecies farm in which the cow manure fertilizes the corn and chickens keep the bugs at bay. Organic farms can be big, and some raise monoculture crops. Companies that dominate the organic food market sell organic berries or vegetable produce nationwide and year-round coming from many farms located in several states and even in other countries like Mexico, Canada, Chile, and Argentina.

The organic produce you buy at your local supermarket probably was not grown by a small family operation, tending each crop using farm-generated fertility (such as manure) to maintain soil fertility. Most likely it wasn't grown by a woman owner-operator or person of color either. But women and workers of color dominate our farm labor scene. Access to land and other agricultural resources is a huge barrier in all kinds of farming, including organic. The low price margins that mega-organic farms can thrive on make competition stiff for other farmers. (I discuss the efficiency advantages of large-scale farms in a later section.)

Another example of weaknesses in the federal organic program—here, a failure to protect as intended—surfaced in my own neighborhood a few years ago. Organic rules prohibit chemical fertilizers but allow the use of manure—even if it comes from large, nonorganic dairies. An organic farm in my region applied manure from a neighbor's dairy, then noticed that many of its broadleaf plants—a majority of its crops—were dying. The problem showed up on other organic farms, too. Throughout the whole county, about 60% of the broad-leafed vegetables on organic farms died that season. Eventually it was discovered that the "next generation" herbicide aminopyralid, produced by Dow AgroSciences, had been applied to control thistle on pastures where that neighbor's dairy cows grazed. But the herbicide remained active even after digestion by the cows and fermentation in manure piles. When the herbicide-contaminated manure was used on the organic crops, the herbicide killed them. So much for those regulations ostensibly protecting organic farmers.

I know it sounds like I am bashing "certified organic"—I like to think of it as questioning. For one thing, the criteria for what qualifies a product to be certified organic (no pesticides, irradiation, or genetic engineering) don't go far enough. But, at the same time, I am grateful for the no–genetic engineering rule. It means that plants or animals whose DNA has been altered, reworked, or reorganized in a laboratory setting are not allowed. This would include, for example, corn plants genetically engineered to resist the chemical glyphosate, used in the weed killer Roundup. Some controversial work and reporting (referenced in the Notes) shows that glyphosate in our diet (ultimately, from the use of weed killers on food plants) may carry a carcinogenic risk; not surprisingly, Monsanto's and Bayer's websites suggest otherwise. Of course, it's not just organic farmers who stay clear of the chemical—but they're the only ones we know for sure are not using it.

Again, we can turn to self-sustaining farms as a potential way forward. Organic farmers who have to import manure are at a disadvantage: there's no way to regulate where that manure comes from, and it's hard for the farmers themselves to be sure. The advantage goes to farmers who can rely mostly on their own farm-generated soil fertility in a more integrated system. Later in this section I'll mention the farm of Scott Meyers and Brigit Waring, who use rotational grazing and cover crops to meet all of their farm's fertility needs. Big monoculture farms can't do this, but farmers who work hard to foster connections with their crops, animals, and land can build their own mini agricultural webs, creating food in a balanced self-contained system right where they live.

Farms where this can happen are often small farms, not the large megascale operations that many types of modern agriculture are trending toward. And small farms *can* thrive. Farmers like the Staps, the Honcoops, and Meyers and Waring—discussed later in this section—are making it happen. Products like theirs don't come close—at least not yet—to dominating the market. But, the market *is* changing. People don't want to eat only megafarmed meat, dairy, and produce anymore. The question is, how FoodWISE are the alternatives we're choosing?

The connection that these small-scale farmers have with their communities—and what it suggests about the value and quality of the food—is increasingly desired by consumers. Quality is, of course, a difficult (albeit subjective) word to define—which plenty of researchers and journalists alike have tried to do. As I mentioned in the Introduction, quality refers to flavor (and smells and textures) of uncontaminated and unadulterated foods. The dilemma for consumers is how to know whether that connection is there when shopping in the grocery store. For many, "organic" is the most useful shorthand label. But how much does that label actually say?

Organic might actually not have much to do with the all-important connection between farmer and consumer that lets us be active, knowledgeable participants in our agricultural web. Organic has become so corporate and industrialized that an organization called the Cornucopia Institute arose to work on "economic justice for the family-scale farming community," with an emphasis on local and organic food. The Cornucopia Institute aims to inform the public about what's behind the organic label on the food they're buying. With some searching you can get information from Cornucopia on mega-farm organic producers like Seeds of Change, Cascadian Farm, Muir Glen, Spectrum Organics, Boca Foods, Horizon, Odwalla, and Morningstar Farms.

I admit, I appreciate the convenience of mega-farm organic greens—it's there in the store, it's washed. And at least I know that municipal sewage sludge was not used as a fertilizer, nor were the products irradiated at some step of processing. Yes, it's not mine, or my farmers market friends', and it may be far from local. On the other hand, I recognize that it is a luxury to be able to buy local at a farmers market. For people who can't, Safeway's local organic still supports a WISEr food culture than Amazon-delivered Dole Food Company might. Again, it's a question of what's important to you, *and* what you can reasonably do. Our mantra should be: stop—think—then act.

On balance, I'd rather buy a Honeycrisp from a local farm that I know than an organic Braeburn apple from New Zealand, even if my neighbor isn't certified organic. A local farm that might use some chemical sprays on its apples, or that just can't afford official organic certification, fits in better with my idea of FoodWISE. Think about the environmental impact generated from shipping apples halfway around the world. Some observers question the resiliency of relying on such international transport, although the extent of that environmental impact is contested.

Food decisions *are* often about connection—being connected to the place where you are, and directly supporting the best practices you can. What I call "true blue" is often better than "global green"; buying that imported apple just makes me think of how many small, local farmers here I'm helping put out of business. My local apple orchard or dairy farm contributes to the local economy. That, in part, pays for my kids' public high school. We're all connected, and the sooner we start actively cultivating the connection, the closer we'll get to a sustainable agricultural future.

The connection to community is a major part of my FoodWISE choices. Admittedly, local isn't everything. Communities consisting of small-scale farms may themselves be producing significant amounts of pollution. But the chances that such pollution is visible, and known, are greater. Relishing the fresh produce we can enjoy from our local farms, as well as questioning the farming practices producing it, are possible when we know the farm and farmer where we get our food. If a good chunk of my county community is female or Latina (which it is) or Native American, then I get very interested in why I don't see more of those faces at farmers markets in my county. I then support as best I can beginning farmer programs (called "farm incubators") that develop a more diverse farming community where I live.

EFFICIENCY AND SUSTAINABILITY?

It makes sense that the whole food system will be more sustainable if we can produce more food while using less land and water and expending less money, labor, energy, or whatever input you care to measure. And, in fact, some of the big efforts that have increased farming efficiency over past decades *have* made certain components of farming more sustainable. We need to recognize, however, that the primary impetus for many new developments has been less virtuous: a search for increased profits, even at the expense of toxic chemicals and dismantled farm communities, has often been behind new efficiencies.

Efficiency: The Green Revolution

An accelerated drive for greater production—touted as an effort to feed the growing world, but also motivated by the constant drive for more profits from greater efficiencies—produced the famed Green Revolution in the 1960s (and before). New chemical pesticides and seeds developed by researchers and disseminated by the agribusiness industry led to a boom in productivity, increasing yields especially of rice and wheat. This evolution of our food system was directed and supported in the United States by farm policies and programs that typically promoted intensification of cultivation and production for export. Agriculture's share of US exports increased, and our national balance of payments (basically, the difference between how much we earn for our manufactured and agricultural goods and services that we export, and how much we owe for what we import) improved. This has all been good for the US economy—and for commercial agriculture's bank accounts. However, this production has mostly been from ever-larger-scale farms and processors. As we'll see, this mega-scale agriculture lacks an element—resilience—that might make the future of US agriculture a bit less rosy than its past.

Efficiency: Regional Crop Specialization

US agriculture is clearly efficient in terms of land use. The latest information from the USDA's Economic Research Service (ERS) reports that, as of 2012, 17% of the nation's land area was used for crop farming, and 34% was used as grassland, rangeland, and grazed forestland for grazing livestock. So, from a total land area of about 2.3 billion acres, about 50% of US land is in some form of agricultural use. It's not a higher percentage thanks to intensification—a heavy reliance on chemical additives for plants and many kinds of confined livestock operations. Intensification of inputs and farming methods means more product from a unit of land, with theoretically lower costs.

Another facet of efficiency is regional specialization—growing what the soil, water, climate, support services, and transportation of a region are suited for. There's a reason why carrots are grown in California and dairy cattle raised in Wisconsin.

Our western states are full of grazing beef cattle that are "finished" in feedlots. The Northwest grows much of the potatoes for our French fries, the Southeast our peanut oil and butter, and sugar—Hawaii and our southern states specialize in genetically engineered (GE) sugar beets, which also grow in the heartland and the West. The results of this drive toward greater efficiency from greater size differ in various parts of the country.

Just how big is a large-scale farm? The USDA has its own definitions, but one way to look at this is to consider the average size of a wheat farm in

Kansas, a sweet potato farm in Arkansas, a carrot operation in California, or a dairy farm in Washington state. Any farm that's substantially bigger than the state average is probably going to be large-scale.

Efficiency: Mega-Scale Agriculture Outcompetes

For many of us, the word "farm" still conjures up an image of a big red barn with a couple of cows, free-running chickens, some fields of crops—all cared for by one dedicated family. That would be small-scale farming, or at least one version of it. Nowadays, though, those farms don't provide much of our food.

In reality, most commercial agriculture production comes from very large-scale farms—they're also called mega-farms—with hundreds or thousands of acres of vegetables, or with hundreds or thousands of one kind of animal packed in a confined area. The simplest reason for the dominance of large farms is efficiency: the economies of scale in operations, the wide range of crop support programs and land use subsidies for larger farms, and the easier access to, and heavy use of, debt financing for equipment purchases and cropping operations. As a general rule, it's cheaper (i.e., more efficient) in economic terms to make a product in a large operation. This ignores, however, some of the key elements of the FoodWISE approach, like community support and ultimately environmental, social, and—in terms of farm debt burdens—economic sustainability.

Before we look more at how efficiencies work in agriculture, let's step aside for a moment and consider the confusing data on "small" family farms. Are small family farms more—or less—important than they used to be in the United States: what's the trend? Indeed, that's a good question. Before the last survey (known as The Agricultural Resource Management Survey), the USDA changed the definition of what constitutes a small family farm. As a result, the percentage of farms classified as "small family" has stayed about the same (87%–90%), over the past fifteen to twenty years—the real change has been in the shift to production by larger farms.

First, a few basic definitions from the USDA: A "farm" is "any place from which $1,000 or more of agricultural products were sold." A "family farm" is "any farm where the majority of the business is owned by the operator and individuals related to the operator."

The first change in definition was the criteria for farm type in relation to sales. A small farm used to be one with less than $250,000 in sales; now the cutoff is $350,000. A midsize family farm has income between $350,000 and $999,999; a large family farm has income over $1,000,000 but less than $5,000,000; and a very large family farm has income over $5,000,000. Non-family farms are not classified by amount of sales. The second change was what counts as farm income, with the effect of now reclassifying many "larger" farms as "small."

The recent situation with farm types, as reported by the USDA's ERS, was that in 2015 small family farms made up 90% of all US farms, operating on 48% of the farmland, and accounting for 24% of overall farm production. The 6% of farms classified as midsize family farms operated on 23% of the acreage and accounted for 23% of production. The 3% of farms classified as large-scale family farms also operated on 23% of the acreage but accounted for 42% of production. The 1% of all farms that were non-family operated on 6% of the farmland and accounted for 11% of US agricultural output. So, the USDA reports that the number of small family farms has stayed about the same for the past two decades, but that's partly because the definition of "small" changed to include more farms.

A slightly different picture is given by another USDA report issued in 2019. It says that the total number of farms declined between 2012 and 2017; only very small farms (sales less than $2,500) and very large ones (sales over $5,000,000) increased in number. Those very large farms accounted for 1% of farms but 35% of all sales. Small farms (sales of $50,000 or less) accounted for 76% of farms but 3% of sales.

What should we make of all this? We will talk more about it later, but a couple of takeaways are that the United States has a great many small- and medium-sized family farms, operating on most of the farmland, but their numbers are shrinking; and that the few, very large farms dominate production. Clearly, farming resources are being concentrated across a small number of big operators.

I must point out that this really is a FoodWISE moment (which I give more examples of in the science section of Part 2). Here we have a whole lot of information on important topics with big implications for how we act. How do we dig into it to understand what it really means? How do we apply our own judgment? As I say elsewhere, we need to: stop—think—then act. We need to understand information presented to us, and think critically about it and about the interpretations and conclusions that are presented with it. In this case, do you think the USDA definitions of family farm size adequately capture the real picture? To me it looks like they're serving to cover up a decline in small family farms.

Back to efficiencies.

Efficiencies of scale also operate in other kinds of agribusiness in the overall agricultural web, namely for suppliers, transporters, processors, and marketers. The clear trend is that both farms and these support businesses are consolidating and getting bigger and bigger.* Here in the United States the pattern has been consolidation by purchase of smaller farms and companies into larger conglomerates with high degrees of specialization, and centralized production and warehousing. According to the Internal Revenue Service, such concentration takes advantage of federal tax incentives. Further, the increasing size of US-based global agribusinesses is part of the reason that most current growth in US agriculture comes from international market expansion.

However, this growth weakens community resilience by reducing the diversity and scale of food sources. Smaller agribusiness operations face heavy competition from large firms in pricing, and therefore suffer declining profit margins.

Impacts on small farms have been a concern of mine for some time. Years back, I became particularly interested in the history of how labor, profitability, social consciousness, and community structure were changing as farming changed. I parlayed these studies into a book (with Prof. Charles C. Geisler) researching the social consequences of agricultural technologies. A common situation I found was: agricultural technology for the privileged few, and tasteless and standardized food for the masses. The machine harvesting of tomatoes was a particularly important case study in this regard.

I persisted on this track and became something of a research geek, studying subjects as varied as the problems of small-scale tobacco growers, cotton harvesting in Oklahoma, how the introduction of mules to thresh grains in the early 1900s spelled disaster for many small farmers who could not afford mules, and the first inklings of problems with a new field called "bioge-netic technology"—now known as genetic engineering. I saw in the mule-technology case a pattern that continues today: not all farmers can afford the newest technology and so, with each new development, the structure of agriculture—the percentage of large-scale farmers growing a particular percentage of food—changes forever. Farms become bigger and fewer, and the fewer produce more. Farm communities change.

Of course, consumer demand is a big factor in what gets produced—and who is able to do the producing. For a time I probed the consequences of consumer pressure to have vegetables and fruits be uniform in shape and maturity. This drive for standard-sized vegetables led to the increased use of technology for plant breeding and harvesting, resulting in greater production and efficiency but also using less labor. Many farmers could not continue in the face of higher technology costs; their departure changed the structure of vegetable and fruit farming: fewer farmers grow-ing more crops.

The mega-scale farms (some would say "factory" farms) that produce most of our food today consume massive amounts of resources, from fossil fuels to chemical fertilizers, in order to produce massive quantities of prod-ucts that they then ship, on a massive scale, around the world. But then again, some make the case that such economies of scale result in greater efficiencies of energy and other inputs. Nevertheless, there are other con-siderations. All this transport inevitably produces wasted food from spoilage in shipping or storage. Sometimes things go wrong and there's even more wastefulness.

One of my students once was involved with an operation to observe the harvesting of 50,000 birds at a large chicken farm (which raised replacement egg-layers), that left about fifty chickens stranded. The story ended well for a few of these chickens—five, at least, were rescued by my student, who then started her own small chicken farm. Not all overlooked animals are so lucky, though, and when you multiply that forty-five that were left by the number of mega-farms in existence, you begin to get some sense of how much waste factory farming can produce. Because of their volume, the farms themselves can afford the loss. *They* can afford it—but can we?

If you've made it this far on your FoodWISE journey, your answer is probably "no": no, we can't afford the risk of contamination from industrial-scale confinement operations; we can't afford to keep taking more than the earth actually has to give. Then there's that other "no": no, we don't want bland tomatoes! Give us real food produced in a sustainable agricultural web.

There's a vulnerability here as well—if we're growing only three kinds of tomatoes, what happens when a new disease decimates one of them? This is discussed more in the "We Need: Biodiversity" section, but I note here that there is some historical precedent for this concern: a lack of biodiversity in potato varieties played a small role in the severity of the Irish potato famine that began in 1845.

This takes us back to the crucial idea of resilience. Not only does less variety mean losing all those delicious, complex tastes that tomatoes can produce—a loss I myself mourn—it also means a higher risk of losing our flavorful tomatoes altogether. If we want an agricultural future, we need biodiversity. As Cary Fowler notes in a TED talk, without the rich genetic mix that evolution has already provided from its vibrant array of adaptations and modifications, we risk losing entire species.

That's certainly how I feel. And a great many farmers out there share this feeling. Across the country, and certainly in my own corner of it, small farmers are making it their mission to grow food in ways that affect the earth far less, while offering a more diverse and tastier product. Resilience is key for these farmers as they figure out ways to stay afloat in a market glutted with cheap imported food. From specialty dairy products to rotational grazing, they have found ingenious ways to keep their small farms not only alive, but thriving.

Small farms (which include, in my general view, anything smaller than mega-scale) are important—ecologically, economically, and culturally. They are the foundation of rural communities, and the origin of many agrarian populists who have fought for policies that protect all scales of farming. I especially value the close connection most small-scale farmers have with their land and plants and animals.

Small farms also keep landscapes as open space (and this is critically important) and retain a diversity of habitats. Although farms of all sizes do preserve open space, small farms tend to have more complexity and provide more ecological functions than very large farms, while avoiding the environmental impacts of large expanses of monoculture.

Open space has all sorts of benefits. For one, losing open space to urbanization (roads, housing, shopping centers, factories) radically changes the character of a place. Many towns and cities all over the United States still have small farms and pockets of rural land on their fringes, adding immeasurably to the character and livability of those communities. Losing agricultural open space to urbanization has local and even regional environmental impacts. These include increased air pollution from vehicles and industry. Further, urbanization is synonymous with an increase in pavement and asphalt roads and sidewalks; these "impervious"-to-water surfaces result in greater stormwater runoff that then pollutes fish habitat (as happens with salmon streams in the Northwest). The importance of open space is widely recognized: its preservation is frequently a major objective of state and local land use planning.

Around the country, there's still some room for small farms that aren't trying to compete with the big enterprises. But it is in mega-agriculture's economic interest to crowd out everybody else—and those most affected are the most vulnerable, with the least financial resources—in the race for top efficiency. Fewer, but bigger, farms—which means less choice for consumers in terms of where we get our food.

Efficiencies in Support Industries, Processing, and Marketing

The consolidation and increase in size we see in farms is mirrored in the transport, distribution, retail, and marketing sectors of the agricultural web. For example, Kroger is the biggest supermarket chain in the world (operating under brands such as Ralphs, Dillons, King Soopers, and Fred Meyer), with $105 billion in sales. Second is Albertsons (with regional chains such as Safeway and Tom Thumb, and $57 billion in sales). Kroger is also the second-largest overall retailer in the world, well behind number one: Walmart, itself a major food store, with $375 billion in total sales in 2017. Walmart's influence is great. See an informative 2007 article published in *Journal of Private Enterprise* on Walmart's influence on local employment.

Big farms and agribusinesses certainly dominate food sales and support services. Mega-agribusiness companies such as Cargill, Nestlé, Monsanto/ Bayer, Conagra, and Archer Daniels Midland work hard to corner specialty markets, while mass-producing consumer products at low prices to out-compete others in those markets. A case in point is Chicken McNuggets from McDonald's, part of the industrial meat complex (discussed later).

Our industrial-scale meat production is itself made possible by the mega-scale growing of soybeans, mainly in the United States, Brazil, and Argentina. Soybean meal accounts for 75% of protein in compounded livestock feeds worldwide. Soymeal is the main source because of its high crude protein content and balanced amino acids, and dominates especially in Europe where meat and bone meal are banned in feeds.

As fast-food chains compete with low prices to sell burgers and chicken, they press their meat suppliers for lower prices. These meat processors, in turn, press the farmers for lower prices. Economies of scale through growth and consolidation result at every stage.

Big poultry "integrators" like Tyson and Perdue manage all aspects of chicken production. They are vertically integrated, from breeding to marketing. They contract out production, from egg to broiler-sized chicken, to a network of farms—now mostly in the American south—that are constantly pressured to do business more cheaply. This industry-wide drive for efficiency does give us fatter, plumper chickens that grow faster—and a food that is cheap. Enter Chicken McNuggets.

McDonald's McNuggets were a creative meat alternative to corn-fed beef, addressing media-driven health concerns about red meat and fat, as well as consumer demand for cheap food. McDonald's mechanically separated chicken meat, shaped into bite-sized pieces, breaded, deep fried, frozen, reheated, and served with processed dipping sauces, entered the world of fast food in 1983. What it isn't is Whole. It is a highly processed product that bears little resemblance to the chicken that people ate even a few decades ago. But this iconic fast food certainly has done well. McDonald's rapidly became the world's second largest seller of chicken.

Efficiencies in raising chickens have led to what can only be called factory farms: animals confined under strictly controlled conditions. It fact, it was my concerns about factory farming in England, while I was a student there in 1974, that originally set me on my path of studying food.

Big institutions don't have to be driven only by efficiency, however. Just as with farming, there are FoodWISE ways of operating at every stage, through processing, marketing, and ultimately getting food onto our plates. For example, while institutional dining services are big food consumers, they are also places where we can find innovative and responsible approaches.

The University of Montana's (UM) Dining Services, under successive directors, aims to serve food that is not only tasty and nutritious, but also seasonal, fresh, and sustainable. Local is key. UM Dining Services collaborates with the Western Montana Growers Co-op, the Mission Mountain Food Enterprise Center, and many other local providers. They bring in food from over twenty counties in Montana, and feature their food-producing partners (aka farmers) on the Dining Services website.

The "Shared Values and Guiding Principles" statement for UM Dining is broad, and includes considerations of nourishment ("We serve wholesome, high quality, and nutritious food"), sustainability ("We commit to local, regional, and global environmental stewardship through sustainable business practices and agricultural economic development in Montana through the UM Farm to College Program"), and diversity ("We respect and celebrate the contributions, rights, and dignity of our diverse employees and guests").

To me, that all sounds FoodWISE.

If you want to dive deeper into the problems besetting our agricultural web, there are many gripping and informative critiques of our current economic/political food system—driven to produce the largest volume at the lowest cost but leaving integrity and the future of the planet out of the mix. Early on, Paul Roberts had given one of the most thorough critiques, along with Harriet Friedmann, Marion Nestle, Michael Pollan, and Eric Schlosser. Steve Ettlinger deconstructed Twinkies, and Gary Taubes carbohydrates, meanwhile Friedman, Nestle, Pollan, and Schlosser, took on whole systems. This array of viewpoints ranges from impressive investigative reporting, to academic articles, to nonprofit advocacy. Academic Julie Guthman adds a postmodern spin, questioning the loss of diversity of farmer and farm, and arguing that that's not an accident. At the end of the day, we're still trying to figure out what to eat.

MEAT

Meat farming and meat consumption invite many questions. Is meat farming/ eating sustainable? Does meat farming cause disproportionate levels of global warming? Does the rearing of animals for meat deprive wild animals of habitat and the world of wilderness? For most of us, eating meat means eating confinement-raised livestock (at least in terms of their "finishing"): are the animals raised and processed humanely? Is killing animals (mostly two- and four-legged ones, but also fish and shellfish) ethical? What gives us humans the right to take a life to feed another life?

Ethical concerns, and questions about meat eating as a waste of food resources, are certainly valid. I think the conclusions and the answers are along the lines of, "Yes, sometimes ... and, maybe sometimes, no."

As we try to sort out the answers for ourselves, at the least we should keep in mind that many well-meaning and thoughtful people are working in the agricultural web on all sides of these issues. Whatever our own stance, let's maintain empathy for the chicken farmer and beef rancher and butcher and try to understand their daily work and their perspectives, as well as for the vegetable farmer and the vegetarian and the herbalist. We're all just working to do the best we can, and we're all just trying to figure it out.

To understand meat production, we need to understand a bit about the physiology of plants and the animals themselves, particularly ruminants like cattle. Ruminants can digest carbohydrates that we can't, which makes them particularly well suited to convert plant protein into animal protein. Nutrients are more concentrated in seeds than in grass blades and stems, so more cattle can be raised on a smaller area and grow quicker when they are fed grain rather than just hay—hence, feedlots. Today, industrialization of farming means grain-fed feedlot operations: chicken in Brazil, dairy in California, pork in the southeast United States. World demand for more meat at lower cost drives mega-scale farming. Increasingly, it is grains and legumes (soybeans, pulses, other beans) that are feeding the world's livestock.

Of course, some of the feed given to animals is from what might be called alternative foods: by-products of the vegetable oil, sugar, beet pulp, grain, or even citrus, fruit, almond, and cotton industries. Similarly, useful livestock by-products—especially manure—should be factored into efficiency calculations and feed conversion ratios. However, in reality many potentially useable by-products are just waste: I have seen thousands of sheepskins in upstate New York sent to landfills.

In other developed countries, mega-scale farming is also the mode. For example, over 60% of Britain's imported pork is from huge farms in Denmark, the Netherlands, and Germany. Among the controversial practices typical of such industries is the heavy use of antibiotics, with vast numbers of pigs being administered antibiotics when just a few animals become infected, although the European Union is putting more restrictions on such use.

The wide administration of antibiotics may well be resulting in resistant strains of diseases. Similarly, the vast, concentrated amounts of animal wastes from such operations lead to many environmental and health concerns. Some waste is turned into fertilizer or biogas, but much of it ends up in manure lagoons or other waste disposal sites. Another issue to note is the welfare of livestock as they are transported. Scholar Michael Appleby has done valuable work on the subject. When transport concerns are combined with broader animal welfare and ethical issues, it's hard to see how mega-scale feedlot production and slaughter are sustainable.

Much has been written about large confinement chicken operations in the United States but also around the world—operations of 500,000 to a million in Thailand, Colombia, and China. Chickens often are raised in huge factory farms: confined, dosed with growth hormones and antibiotics, slaughtered at six to eight weeks or less, and bred for oversized breasts (with the unbalanced growth leading to problems in walking). The dominant meat breed—the Cornish cross—is also used by a lot of small-scale growers because it does grow quicker, eats less feed in its shorter life, and consumers have come to think it's what chicken should be like. It is sometimes referred to as the Frankenchicken. I will admit that my family, too, raised this breed one year, but then we went back to a tastier (to my mind), although somewhat less efficient, heritage variety.

Part of the meat conundrum is the high demand we create. In the United States, we eat a lot of meat—an estimated 222 pounds of red meat and poultry per person in 2018, up from the previous several years and a new record. We want a lot of meat, and we want it cheap.

One way to avoid many of the problems with meat from livestock, although it hasn't gone mainstream yet, is to get meat from wildlife. It's the hunter-gatherer alternative, about as natural as you can get. Perhaps hunting for food will catch on with people concerned about whole, natural food.

GENETICALLY ENGINEERED (GE) PLANTS AND ANIMALS

Farms and other food industries would make more profit if the living organisms—the plants and animals—at the foundation of the business would just do their jobs better. They should grow faster, be more resistant to pests and diseases and drought, and do clever things like be resistant to herbicides used to kill their competing weeds. Enter genetic engineering (GE), which we have defined as plants or animals whose DNA has been altered, reworked, or reorganized in a laboratory setting. I've already mentioned one application of this technology, the production of food plants resistant to the herbicide glyphosate, as a potential problem for our food supply.

Are warmer temperatures extending insects' breeding periods, causing a spike in pests? For companies such as Monsanto/Bayer and DuPont, this problem translates into "we need a new kind of plant that's more pest resistant!" An early GE corn, for example, was manufactured with material from the bacterium *Bacillus thuringiensis,* which secretes a natural pesticide, thus producing a plant that can kill its own insect pests.

Perhaps the most well-known GE example is the one I've mentioned in the Introduction—Roundup Ready corn and soybeans. Monsanto patented the molecule glyphosate for use as a herbicide in 1970, and first marketed it in 1974 in its herbicide Roundup, also patented. The German drug and crop chemical maker Bayer completed purchase of Monsanto in June 2018 and is dropping the Monsanto name from its products. I'll continue to refer to "Monsanto," because that was part of the history of certain chemicals discussed in this book. "Roundup Ready" is the trademark for Monsanto/Bayer's patented genetically engineered crop seeds that are resistant to glyphosate. Since the patent on glyphosate expired almost two decades ago, numerous other chemical companies have produced and marketed glyphosate. Roundup kills pretty much any plant it touches—except Monsanto/Bayer's own proprietary GE crops. This means that farmers can spray weeds with no negative effect on their crops. However, it also can mean that every other plant in the vicinity dies, including on neighboring farms if the herbicide drifts on the breeze.

Other problems have been raised in scientific and popular literature, including contamination of organic crops by pollination from GE crops, and the question of what we are ingesting when we eat that sprayed corn. Further, as was totally predictable, weeds, with repeated exposure, are adapting and evolving resistance to glyphosate. New and more powerful herbicides will be needed—with implications for natural systems and human health. Glyphosate itself has been scrutinized for years, and there's increasing evidence that exposure to it is much worse for our health than we were told, including raising the risk of some cancers.

But apart from these serious problems, for me one of the biggest arguments against large-scale use of GE seeds—such as corn, canola, cotton, soy, and sugar beets—is its effect on the structure of agriculture: who produces what. GE crops help big farmers get bigger and contribute to squeezing out smaller and even midsize farms, farms that are already economically vulnerable. Apart from higher yields, these GE technologies give mega-farms more predictability about their harvests and, in this sense, may lessen the financial uncertainties they face.

As part of this pressure, proprietorship issues plague some farmers, including those who didn't buy the patented GE seed but are accused of (and sometimes sued for) using the patented seed, because windblown GE pollen alighted on their fields. There's also the question of who owns the genetic material from which all these new discoveries come. Can the genes and their patented traits in these seeds be considered a form of scientific intellectual property?

But at the crux of all this is the big-gets-ever-bigger agricultural juggernaut.

Given the many controversies over GEs, it's understandable that consumers want to know whether there are GEs in the food they buy. From our FoodWISE perspective, a relevant part of the acronym is the "I" for "Informed." Without required labeling for GEs, the only way to know if a food is GE-free is to buy certified organic—and even then, in some cases, organic farmers may use GE seeds if no others are available. Without labeling for GEs, the ability of consumers to vote with their dollars to influence the sustainability of agriculture—from both an environmental and a social perspective—is greatly reduced.

LABOR

Big is good for efficiency in several ways when it comes to the use of labor— at least from the perspective of the larger farms. Bigger agricultural enterprises can afford more machines to do the work with less labor. They may have greater bargaining power in setting wages and other compensation for the smaller labor forces they do have. The labor force is nevertheless essential, especially in fruit and vegetable production.

US agricultural businesses, both farms and processors, depend on temporary migrant labor, mainly from Mexico and Latin America, or recent immigrants. These farm workers perform labor that few US-born workers want to do at the same wage. Tomato-picking is backbreaking labor. Dealing with animals, meat, and waste in processing plants is hard and, to many, unpleasant. Dairy workers put in odd shifts, including through the night. Raspberry-picking requires most daylight hours in the field during peak season. Tending and picking brassicas—kale, broccoli, cauliflower, and brussels sprouts and their seeds—also require long hours in the field.

Most hired farm labor is for work on fruit, vegetable, and horticultural crops—collectively referred to as FVH commodities. Large FVH farms are concentrated in California, followed by Florida, Texas, and Washington. The labor for FVH crops in California is 93% foreign-born; FVH workers in the United States (excluding California) are 83% foreign-born. Animal operations, particularly dairy, also count on a relatively high percentage of such labor.

The unsettled status of national policy on immigrant agricultural labor means great uncertainty for farmers and processors—as well as for the people themselves who perform the work. As labor continues to be a substantial percentage of farm cash costs, operations relying on it remain vulnerable. No one knows at this time whether agricultural labor, the way it works now, is sustainable.

Another aspect of labor is more clear-cut: what are the terms of work, namely wages, other forms of compensation, and working and living conditions? An equitable food system following the FoodWISE approach requires that these terms be fair to the workers. Labor costs can be a big part of farm or processor expenses, and, as with most businesses, finding mutually acceptable terms of employment affecting wages and revenues can be difficult. Yet, sustainability requires knowledgeable, capable, and maybe long-term workers, so that balance has to be found.

The same issues apply to food businesses on up the chain, perhaps most strikingly at the retail level where efficiencies drive practices that don't fit our FoodWISE standards. At the US and world's top grocery chain/retailer, Walmart, I don't care if the cereal costs $2 if the person at the checkout counter is not making a living wage, because that person and that person's wages are also part of the agricultural web.

Resilience in agriculture necessarily includes a sustainable supply of labor—which basically translates into "well-enough paid, well-enough compensated." Right now, a willing labor force exists—but that force is under threat. Any deportation policies targeting agricultural workers would greatly affect the agricultural web, particularly in places like my home state of Washington, which is a major fruit grower and thus heavily dependent on foreign-born labor. Analysts, even conservative ones at the Washington Policy Center, are looking at what's happening with labor policy as it becomes increasingly clear that, without migrant labor, we won't have farms.

For several decades, Phillip L. Martin of the University of California has written on progressive immigration reform to ensure that we still have people to work our farms. This means facilitating a path for authorized and unauthorized migrant workers to become US residents, and a shift from current practices that force farmers to rely on thousands of unauthorized foreign-born workers—who are increasingly at risk of deportation if they make it into the United States at all.

Further, with "unauthorized" status comes substantial risk and uncertainty in the lives of the workers. With no Social Security benefits, no guarantees of education, and no legal resources available, these workers live on the edge in a way few native-born US citizens can imagine. The seasonal nature of agricultural labor only increases that uncertainty.

A workforce in constant fear of illness, unemployment, or deportation hardly spells resilience for the farms these workers currently keep afloat. Clearly, if we want to keep growing food, we're going to have to find a way to keep our labor force.

It all comes back to resilience. Just as we need to maintain healthy soil in order to grow food, to build connections between farmers and communities, to support farms that don't rely on vulnerable off-farm sources of fertility, so do we also need workers. Eliminating 20% of our farm workers—which is what legal-only workers translates into—means billions of dollars of losses, especially on mega-scale but also small-scale farms. It's just possible (although hard to imagine with FVH crops) that some of those mega-farms could handle the setback, but smaller farms are vulnerable—and, as we've seen, it's those smaller farms that any FoodWISE consumer needs to keep alive.

A FoodWISE approach considers a farm's place in the greater social and economic web and takes the long view to do what is necessary for labor to be sustainable. Wages can be where a farm looks to cut costs as it struggles financially to stay above water. Every region has its own challenges: in New York, for example, "There is almost unbelievable pressure in the Hudson Valley to develop real estate, to pay workers bottom-low wages, to work the bottom line," says M. B. Ryan of Breezy Hill and Stone Ridge orchards.

Ryan considers the "social ecosystem" to be just as important as the natural world her apples grow in. Whole for her extends not only to the fresh fruit, cider, and apple pies, but also to the families who helped pick and make them. "My livelihood rises and falls" with the families who work for her, she says.

A Cornell University graduate with a degree in pomology, Ryan has been in the business for three and a half decades. Competition for her products seems to grow ever more intense, but she has found a way to keep her head above water, clocking many long hours of direct marketing and maintaining a well-compensated labor force.

CLIMATE CHANGE

It seems hard to argue that there is any bigger threat to the long-term sustainability of our food system than climate change. Climate affects our whole environment and how we use it; as climate changes, so will the ways we use the world around us. Moreover, the agricultural web—farming and transportation, in particular—has played a part in causing the climate to change.

Climate change is all about increased human-caused greenhouse gases in the atmosphere. Animals breathe in oxygen and breathe out carbon dioxide. Plants take in carbon dioxide and, after extracting the carbon for growth through photosynthesis, emit oxygen. When both animals and plants die, a lot of the carbon in their bodies gets stored, generally speaking, in the ground. When the amount of carbon-dioxide-in and carbon-dioxide-out remains more or less in balance, earth's atmosphere maintains its approximate prehistorical composition of gases. Which is good, because the earth needs to radiate back out to space some of the heat it receives from the sun or its temperature will rise, yet carbon dioxide (and other gases like methane, a product of organic decomposition) blocks some of that re-radiation of heat. When the concentration of these gases reaches a certain level, they, in effect, turn the atmosphere into a kind of greenhouse.

The composition of the atmosphere in pre-industrial ages usually made just the right kind of greenhouse: not too warm, not too cold. With no atmosphere, the earth would be as cold as the moon. It's a precarious balance.

What has happened in recent decades is that too much carbon dioxide and other gases in the atmosphere are blocking too much re-radiation and causing the earth to heat up. The simple explanation is that more carbon dioxide has been emitted into the atmosphere since the start of the Industrial Revolution, and is currently accelerating from the combustion of fossil fuels (coal, oil)—while the carbon stored in living vegetation has simultaneously been reduced by other changes like reduction of the world's forests. Many other processes are involved in global warming as well—the not-yet-well-understood role of oceans in storing and circulating heat and gases, and the release of gases from "sinks" like permafrost as arctic areas warm.

Farming worldwide will have to change as climate changes. Those changes include rainfall increases in some places and decreases elsewhere, rising growing temperatures for crops, unpredictable pest and disease response, intensively cultivated regions becoming uninhabitable due to coastal flooding, and so on. US farmers know this, and are scrambling to adapt. An article about eleven common crops that are being affected by climate change shows the magnitude of the problem even within our own country.

Agriculture is partly responsible. Burning fossil fuels for electricity, heat, and transportation is the biggest source of carbon dioxide in the United States. Long-distance and global transport of agricultural commodities contribute to this.

Besides the carbon dioxide that livestock respire, a lot of methane—an even more powerful heat-trapping gas than carbon dioxide—is released from the mind-boggling amounts of manure produced in livestock operations. Another very potent greenhouse gas—nitrous oxide—is increasingly released into the atmosphere by the action of soil microbes processing nitrogen from vast amounts of synthetic fertilizers used in farming globally, and also from stored manure. And, importantly, much of the vast areas of carbon-storing forests that are clear-cut worldwide—in the Amazon, in Malaysia, in West Africa—are for food: soybeans, cattle, sugarcane, and palm oil.

A dependable source for climate information is the Climate Impacts Group (CIG) at the University of Washington. (The reliability of sources of useful scientific information is important, and I will talk more about that in Part 2.) The goal of CIG science and policy researchers is to work with decision makers to understand climate science and risks, in order to boost regional climate resilience. The research is multidisciplinary—with scientists from many disciplines, but also interdisciplinary—combining knowledge and approaches from multiple fields to try to come up with better answers to hard questions about climate. This is a winning strategy—we will see this again in Part 2, where we discuss scientists' attempts to answer difficult questions about diet. The group calls this strategy the "intersection of knowledge generation and application." The questions they are investigating are about climate and ecosystem modeling, but also vulnerability assessment—who's likely to be most disadvantaged from climate change impacts, and what are some good strategies for adaptation.

Much of CIG's work is far-reaching. In a 2015 report, *State of Knowledge: Climate Change in Puget Sound,* the scientists identify some of the important long-term changes that can be expected that will affect agriculture.

Reasonable projections for change are essential for planning. How to prepare for such change is under our control. If farmers know what to expect, they can prepare, prioritizing resilience. Colleagues and I at Western Washington University have also mapped out climate change scenarios and impacts as a result of agricultural practices. In our Farm Resilience Project, farmers themselves are thinking about potential disaster scenarios and talking about how they could be resilient and adapt. You can see farmer interviews from this study, an interactive map, and a three-minute film we produced at https://wp.wwu.edu/gigiberardi/resilient-farm-project-2009-current/. In our work, but also elsewhere, the need for partnerships with public agencies at all levels of government is urgent.

Climate is very complex (that's an understatement!) and there are many approaches to trying to predict what will happen, ranging from greenhouse gas scenarios (what happens if our carbon output increases by x amount?) to climate modeling based on global temperature changes (what happens if current trends continue?). Keep in mind, too, that different regions of the earth will experience different changes. Yet from Bill McKibben's anti-carbon campaign group 350.org, to Bob Inglis's RepublicEn, a conservatives-for-climate-change-solutions group, the call for concern and action on all levels is clear. Here in the Northwest, farmers are getting worried.

Just as climate change itself can seem almost impossibly complex, so too can our assessment of how much particular activities—like beef farming or an airplane trip, or particular products like a new car or an apple from Chile—contribute to it. The common way to do this is to figure out something's "carbon footprint," a term I use in this book. It is especially useful when comparing products and activities regarding our human impacts. Many carbon-footprint calculators are available online. But the term's limitations must be recognized.

Basically, "carbon footprint" is an imprecise and inadequate term. "Footprint" signifies impact, and "carbon" refers to the amount of carbon dioxide produced (or its carbon equivalent). But what gets included in the calculation is highly variable, and impacts on climate change from things other than carbon are not included. Furthermore, the full carbon costs of many things are so complex they are virtually impossible to measure, and some that are measurable, like imported bananas, suggest surprisingly low impacts. The difficulties inherent in the term are exhaustively and humorously explored by Mike Berners-Lee in *How Bad Are Bananas?: The Carbon Footprint of Everything*. Gary Adamkiewicz of Harvard University has spoken about the related concept of food miles, as well as how buying "local" might not always be the best option to reduce carbon emissions. Adamkiewicz handles conundrums and nuance well. Local is a good principle, but not necessarily a universal rule, in terms of carbon impacts on the environment.

HOW DO WE GET TO FOODWISE?

Given the current state of our agricultural web—which can look fairly dire—what, then, needs to change to match our FoodWISE ideas? What can we individually (or collectively) do to make our own approach to food more WISE? The answers must be: a number of things—some harder, some easier.

We Need: Small-Scale, Integrated Farms

If it were easier for farm and retail businesses to stay small, more of them would. But economies of scale are hard to beat—whether you're buying seed in bulk or handling thousands of gallons of milk. But part of being FoodWISE is farming ingeniously, with some objectives in mind besides the financial bottom line. It's good for the soul. It's good for the planet. It's good for food.

On many small farms, practical wisdom encourages an entrepreneurial spirit, wanting to do more than the minimum required. Farmers understand the need to balance the restrictions of food safety rules (like the sixty-day minimum aging requirement for raw milk cheeses) with their other aims, like producing the highest flavor. Rules talk needs to be tempered with wisdom talk, like what's needed to achieve the FoodWISE flavor profile of that cheese.

For the "E"—"Experience" and "Empathetic" (the empathy I referred to in the Introduction)—we need to appreciate and sometimes imagine all the hard decisions farmers make and the constraints they face. The kind of demoralizing institutional demands that bear down on farmers are illustrated in a film our university group made, *Our Farms Are at Risk*. The farmers themselves are keenly aware that "big" does not necessarily mean "better." Thinking things through in terms of "resilience" helps in understanding how they manage, and they see and reflect on that themselves in the film.

Efficient often means big, and big usually means specialized. A common way this happens is separating the production of animals from the production of their feed. One business raises chickens, another farm raises the grain to feed them. But integrated, mixed crop/livestock systems are the key to sustainability—at least in terms of having a guaranteed source of soil fertility in the form of manures and composts. Manure from a smaller operation is more manageable; if properly handled (and, of course, there are no guarantees here), it is less likely to escape from a storage lagoon in a big rain, and is easier to use to fertilize the soil (although small-scale operators also need to take caution). Recycling the nutrients by using livestock manure to fertilize crops and pastures is a central part of integrated farming. Integrated farming systems better connect plants with animals.

If a farmer was avoiding chemical fertilizer and animal manures, how else could the fields be fertilized? Cover crops—clover, vetch, rye, spring oats, wheat, barley, and even lentils (as shown in Liz Carlisle's *Lentil Underground*) can contribute fertility. Taking a FoodWISE approach toward an integrated, biological solution may lead us to sorghum-sudangrass: its deep roots are massive, and it provides good habitat for microorganisms and biomass for the soil when decayed. These regenerative land use strategies also create diverse pastures of flowering cover crops that support pollinators: all is integrated.

After all, land and water are where it all starts. The land provides, but only if crops harvested and nutrients removed are replaced with sustainable nutrients and the land itself is not overgrazed. This is the balance that farmers Scott Meyers and Brigit Waring of Lopez Island, Washington, aim for.

Meyers and Waring sell cows but they call themselves grass farmers, not cattle ranchers. About twenty years ago, they moved from the Washington mainland to Lopez Island to farm. An island brings its own particular challenges but their most difficult problems turned out to be the poor quality of the soils. This could have led them to rely on imported feed and chemical soil additives, like so many large-scale farms do. Instead, they assessed what their land was able to give and committed to finding a more sustainable way to farm.

Over the years Meyers and Waring have reclaimed their compacted, overgrazed, seasonally flooded land and turned it into top-grade pasture. They did this by using a combination of rotational grazing, draining excess surface water that can't soak into the clay soils, and taking the cattle off soggy fields during the rainy winter. Rotational grazing is the key, limiting compaction and preventing overgrazing while replenishing nutrients with manure. They also reseed with mixtures that include nitrogen-fixing fodder plants like legumes to bolster the soil's fertility. The upshot is that their cattle are completely pasture-fed.

Farming this way has many challenges. From a situation of too much surface water in typical winters, lately they've experienced several years in a row that have been drier than normal. They have to adapt to this and manage their soils more intensively. This means moving animals around, which takes time and resources.

A prominent exemplar of how to manage such rotational grazing systems is agrarian evangelist Joel Salatin. Salatin is a fervent believer in small-scale farming with pastured animals and rotational grazing. He works a crowd beautifully to convert the audience: manage the grazing, watch the animals, optimize root growth, produce the best possible grass—the only limitations are the farmer's cleverness and time.

The level of intensive management practiced by Meyers and Waring, and by Salatin, gives them a close connection to the food they produce. Such connection would be inconceivable on a mega-scale farm managed for maximum financial efficiency. Integrated farms should be relatively small scale to be FoodWISE.

Small-scale intensive farming invariably takes a lot of effort and attention and often carries big financial risks. Take the Honcoop raspberry operation in Whatcom County, Washington, where I live. Raspberries are big here; the county produced over 72 million pounds of red raspberries in 2018. This amounts to about 90% of the nation's total production of red raspberries destined for the processing market (for freezing and for juice, jam, and other foods), according to raspberry farmer and member of the Board of Directors of the Washington Red Raspberry Commission, Randy Honcoop.

The fertile, temperate landscape also supports numerous insects of different kinds that can destroy the growing canes or the fruit itself: raspberry cane-borer beetles with yellow markings, a metallic blue-black red-necked cane borer, white maggots, the expanding threat of the invasive spotted-wing *drosophila,* and many others. Most large raspberry farms spray pesticides monthly—including chemicals for weed and disease control.

Raspberry farmer Randy Honcoop understands that pesticides devastate any flora or fauna that's not, well, a raspberry. Instead, Honcoop uses a version of Integrated Pest Management (IPM) to control pests on his relatively small farm of about sixty acres, which amount to less than 1% of total Whatcom County red raspberry acreage. Still, it's a lot of investment for him to protect.

In IPM, the amount of pest damage is assessed before any action is taken, and then, ideally, only a minimal treatment is used. IPM practices are targeted at actual pest populations. Some practices are consistent with organic production: cultivating the soil to stop insect growth, cutting out less vigorous canes, using pheromone traps, manually picking beetles off the plants, or releasing beneficial insects like ladybugs in the fields to eat aphids. Other problems can be controlled somewhat with compounds like lime sulfur or copper sulfate.

During both the dormant and growing seasons, Honcoop is out in his berry fields every day scouting for adult insects, larvae, and eggs—and looking for damage. He counts bugs. If his assessments are wrong, he might not apply enough treatment. On the other hand, he doesn't want to apply too much. The sprays are toxic to bees and to his "beneficials" such as ladybugs and praying mantises—and they are expensive, too. He's cautious in using them.

Honcoop is answering for himself the question, what can I do to make it better? He calculates that his pest management approach saves him money in the long term, and he knows it is better for his pollinators, his soil, and the environment in general. But he faces risks with this approach; some miscalculations are inevitable. In two of the past ten years he lost some of his crop by waiting too long to spray. Each season, he gains experience and information to guide him the next year.

Every farm takes something different to succeed. The owners of Twin Brook Creamery in Lynden, Washington, have made crucial business moves that typify how flexible and innovative a small-scale operation can—and must—be.

Debbie and Larry Stap, the farm's owners and operators, had a problem. Declining milk prices and no farming opportunities for younger family members meant their farm wasn't resilient anymore—they couldn't see how they would compete in a market overrun by high-volume-oriented, cheap product. Their solution? Diversify. Give people something new, unlike anything they'd be able to find on supermarket shelves.

Larry Stap is a fifth-generation dairy farmer born and raised in the northwest corner of the United States. For years he sold to the regional milk cooperative, Darigold. But he realized expansion would be necessary to make room for his son-in-law, who wanted to farm as well.

Frankly, there's not a lot of profitable middle ground in US farming—and especially dairy farming, where profit margins are particularly low. Our current agricultural web exerts an economic squeeze on small family farms (defined as those with farm income less than $350,000) and on midsize ones (with farm income between $350,000 and $999,999). As we saw earlier, these farms account for 24% and 23%, respectively, of overall US farm production. In a former era, many of these farms might have been considered "large" family farms and constituted a higher percentage of the total production, but they can no longer compete with the big mega-scale operations. Farmers have to mass-produce in order to bring down overall costs. But what about farmers like the Staps, who want to run a farm that's too big to rely on selling only to small or direct markets, the kind of specialty markets that could be profitable for some small farmers?

They needed to figure out something to give people that those big farms couldn't. That's when they had their inspiration: high-quality milk, in reusable glass bottles. High quality would mean low-temperature, small-vat pasteurization—a more "whole" method of preservation. To get started, Stap moved eighteen of his Jersey cows from the larger dairy into what he called "the penthouse," a dairy barn closer to his house, so he could keep an eye on "his girls."

Jersey milk has a higher protein and fat content than milk from most other breeds, and therefore a richer flavor, which, Stap reasoned, would be preserved by his careful pasteurization. He also decided not to homogenize the milk, further preserving the taste and allowing the relatively high percentage of cream or butterfat to float to the top. Not homogenizing preserves the integrity of the fat globules. Stap wants his milk whole in the truest sense of the word. Even his choice to use glass bottles contributes: glass does not alter the taste of the milk the way cardboard cartons or plastic containers sometimes can.

Stap has expanded the number of milking cows in his "penthouse" to 190—a bigger operation, but still a small dairy by industry standards. He has upgraded his bottling machine to handle seven bottles at a time rather than the previous two (which were capped by hand). Besides selling milk and cream, in the late fall he sells his own eggnog—which is so popular he can't keep it on the shelves, especially in larger Seattle markets.

Stap has intentionally kept the operation small, not only to be economical but to retain cash as part of maintaining the operation's resiliency. If equipment repairs are needed, or if his land floods, he has the cash resources to deal with those challenges. Many of his markets are nearby, and he only takes on as many sales as he can handle given his milk production. Fair wages mean labor costs are high—some are family, some hired. Intensive labor is what makes his operation successful, he figures. He is connected to the process at all points along the way.

Could he get bigger? Would there be a market? Could he use another bottling facility? Yes! "But why?" asks Stap. "That would only be greed."

Twin Brook Creamery is an example of the kind of operation that produces FoodWISE food. The milk is whole: minimally processed and unadulterated. It is not inexpensive, but it is not priced higher than it costs to keep Twin Brook running. Imaginative it is—the Staps were among the first to return to glass bottling and low-temperature vat processing, in an age when other milk, including organic, may be ultra-pasteurized. The Staps' practices are informed and intuitive: they keep the Staps connected with their family and cows. And what they're making is whole food. Their farm is sustainable: they operate within their means, they manage their animals and pasture and water carefully. Financially, they have been able to stay in business a long while and seem like they will continue to do so.

Apart from the food it produces, Twin Brook is also a good example of a successful, responsible, multigenerational, small-scale family farm. The

Staps pay close attention to the economic and regulatory currents swirling around them and work hard to keep their farm's place in the greater agricultural web, even to the extent that the community has financed some of their diversification, in the true meaning of the Latin root for credit, *cred,* as in *credere,* "to believe (in)."

What does Twin Brook Creamery tell us about the future of whole foods? For one thing, that a future exists. The Staps made their farm more Whole, not less, in order to compete in the modern market. Now they can offer consumers higher-quality milk products, produced by pastured cows with favorable fatty acid and protein composition—nutrients our bodies need—as compared to milk from mega-farms with 10,000 or more cows in some western states.

We Need: Biodiversity

For me, tomatoes will always symbolize much that is wrong with modern agriculture—but also some of the pleasures and satisfactions of being myself a small part of alternative systems. Some of you readers have a lot more experience growing tomatoes than I did, even after four years of teaching food courses as a graduate student at Cornell, when, for part of my master's thesis research, I lived with a group of old-order Mennonite organic farmers in central Pennsylvania. Among other crops they grew tomatoes. At harvest time we had literally tons of them in the field. I still remember the backbreaking work of harvesting, and the gummy, sticky residue on the ground (we were all barefoot, feet being easier to clean than shoes), on the plants, and on us. All in sweltering heat. I learned a lot about tomato plant spacing, insect control, and particularly post-harvest losses—most of which were quite smelly.

At about the same time, rural populist (and later Secretary of Agriculture for Texas) Jim Hightower released *Hard Tomatoes, Hard Times.* This report of the Agribusiness Accountability Project on the failure of US land grant colleges to meet the needs of small-scale growers was a well-worded polemic against mega-scale farms. It highlighted wealthy constituencies, racial discrimination, little transparency, and (literally) hard tomatoes as major problems associated with the government-funded agricultural research complex. Hightower used tomatoes as a great example of more widespread, pervasive failures. Bred for tough skin but also poor maturity, those tomatoes were perfect for machine harvesting, thus maximizing profits but minimizing quality of taste, and possibly even nutrition.

When I think of the industrial-style tomatoes Hightower describes next to the tasty "whole food" tomatoes in the Pennsylvania countryside that stained my feet and exploded on my tongue—well, there is no comparison. Anyone who grows her or his own tomatoes can experience firsthand the difference between plants grown hands-on, with all the care and time that that entails, and those grown for the mass market. The Mennonites' soft, juicy tomatoes persist today mostly in people's backyards. Elsewhere, tomatoes are a globalized product tended by economically vulnerable people working in backbreaking positions, high heat, and humidity, with unacceptable living and working conditions—labor organizing here, and actually for much of agriculture, has not been successful.

Just as diversity of farming types contributes greatly to the resilience and therefore sustainability of farming communities in the face of change, so it is for the plants and animals that are the foundation of the food system. Promoting small, integrated farms is a key strategy for farming sustainability; and, similarly, protecting the variety of seeds and livestock breeds is the essence of agricultural biodiversity. We need tasty, soft, hard-to-ship tomatoes, not just hard, practical ones.

There was a time—around the turn of the last century—when the USDA actually handed out seeds to farmers, reportedly millions of packages. Today, free seeds are a thing of the past. Genetic engineering allows a level of ownership and control of access to seeds never before possible in agriculture. Seeds, such as the Roundup Ready varieties we talked about earlier, can have patented traits, making them a form of intellectual property even when the basic raw material (the seed itself) may be owned by another farmer or even another country. Agribusinesses market their engineered seeds on the (often correct) premise that farmers will be willing to pay the higher price of new, hybrid seeds if the purchase is justified by, say, increases in productivity. Critics, though, argue that plant genetic resources are being appropriated, to be turned into, literally, cash crops grown by and for the wealthy. Activist scholars such as Vandana Shiva, and in the United States, Cary Fowler, have investigated and written about issues of property rights in India, Brazil, and elsewhere.

Certainly the world is changing and we do need to make space for new innovations in commercial agriculture. This doesn't have to mean privatization of intellectual property, though; these developments could be made while still protecting the genetic plant resource base, so that it is available for use by any grower or breeder. Collecting, conserving, protecting biodiversity—these are all important parts of ensuring a resilient agriculture, now and for the future.

Consumers can see the importance of agricultural biodiversity in so many ways. Journalist Simran Sethi in *Bread, Wine, Chocolate: The Slow Loss of Foods We Love* talks about the loss of taste diversity: twenty-one kinds of potato chips but only five kinds of potato; or, a handful of kinds of apple in a store when many times more are grown commercially in the United States. Researchers Colin Khoury and colleagues have tried to quantify changes (basically downward) in diversity in the crop species that contribute to global food supply. They have looked at trends over the last fifty years in the abundance and composition of crop species, and the results are daunting.

Best known is the banana problem. We basically eat only one kind of banana: the endangered Cavendish. Genetically old and biologically sterile, this popular forest fruit, selected for having soft fruit without seed, is now highly endangered due to its inability to change, to be resilient. It has no possibility for adaptation. The genetic accident that made it seedless (and tasty, not that these two traits necessarily go together) made it an evolutionary dead end. Before the Cavendish, the Gros Michel was in vogue, but it pretty much died off due to the soil fungus *Fusarium oxysporum*. The Cavendish was resistant but it's not so much anymore, as its diseases and other threats have evolved and changed, but its genetics have not.

So, at the production end of things, loss of biodiversity of crops, of livestock, of fertility sources, of pest controls, of whole farming systems rolls on. One of many programs pushing back is that of Stephen Jones of Washington State University. Jones is a wheat breeder and director of the well-known Bread Lab, itself a think tank and baking laboratory for scientists, farmers, chefs, brewers, and others who want both flavor and nutrition, as well as functionality, from their grains. Stephen Jones and his team are committed to plant breeding specifically for local food systems, and this includes small grains and dry beans.

Moving away from the dominant plant breeding model of today, Jones and others believe that selection of heirloom varieties should be driven by the needs of farmers and chefs and millers—those actually using the grains. Further, Jones is committed to looking at the ethics of plant breeding and correcting how exclusionary the practice has been for decades. This is plant breeding with a heart, focused on preserving what I see as a critical piece to FoodWISE thinking: preserving farming communities by making production innovative, competitive, and economically viable.

The virtues of a nontraditional crop can be seen in what might have been considered the unlikely success of lentils in Montana, a story told by Carlisle in *Lentil Underground*. She relates how graduate school dropout David Oien returned to his 280-acre family farm in what was then grain-dominated eastern Montana to plant a renegade crop: lentils—and organic at that. Fast-forward thirty-five years and Oien and a handful of partners are still growing and assisting others to grow lentils, as well as peas, barley, chickpeas, and spelt through their company Timeless Natural Food. Over the years, Timeless has been a boost to the local economy via expanded employment and farming opportunities. More broadly, the production of lentils and other pulses has continued to expand and become a significant crop sector across the dry plains of the north-central United States and southern Canada.

We Need: Policies That Support Resilience

Journalist and author Paul Roberts says we need to be "thinking" food-system consumers. Academic writer Julie Guthman says we need to understand the workings of the state as much as changing market forces. I say we need to be FoodWISE about how government policies affect the food system.

A lot of agricultural policy uses subsidies as a main mechanism to encourage particular kinds of production. Subsidies aren't necessarily bad. I would be all for subsidies that redress the imbalance of other incentives and promote a more resilient agriculture. Or, from the consumers' point of view, as Julie Guthman advocates, subsidies that "allow all eaters to buy what they want and need."

National agricultural subsidies now come in a variety of guises, from direct crop-support payments to crop insurance. Further, in the 2018 Farm Bill (otherwise known as the Agricultural Improvement Act of 2018), there are relatively few restrictions on subsidy caps (i.e., payments per person, and also payments per extended family members). But such policies and programs support the *stability* of agriculture, the ability to keep doing the same thing into the future—not *innovation and flexibility,* not *resilience.* More money goes into trying to make sure a farmer doesn't lose everything growing soybeans again this year than goes into trying to help find a different way to grow soybeans or a different crop altogether if the climate changes.

For small-scale farmers, the overall market is shaped by the subsidies of their big-business competitors. There needs to be government policy that helps small-scale farmers to be more resilient (although the 2018 Farm Bill makes some strides in this direction) so that big companies do not get all the benefits, and at small farms' expense. Assistance could include support for particular production practices, or inexpensive credit and financing.

It wasn't always like this. The Roosevelt administration took on mega-farming to advocate for agricultural workers, tenant farmers, and small-scale family farmers as part of the Depression-era "New Deal." The wide-ranging Agricultural Adjustment Act of 1933 (reauthorized periodically as the "Farm Bill") was meant to adjust prices by controlling supply through production controls and subsidy payments. But the size of farms was always a concern, and various programs dealt with the disadvantaged smaller-scale farms and the landless. Two agencies of the USDA, the Farm Security Administration (FSA) and the Bureau of Agricultural Economics (BAE), continued through World War II in their efforts to aid landless farmers. At one point the FSA had 800,000 client families, some of its programs at least 20% African American. It established, among other things, networks of grassroots land-use planning committees from a broad population base, working with scientists. Another program to help smaller farmers and the landless was the Rural Rehabilitation program of the FSA, which provided loans, grants, and technical assistance to tenants, sharecroppers, and other struggling farmers. Other successful programs included group medical and dental plans, and established farm labor standards for migrant labor camps built in California. Tens of thousands may have benefited—but millions more did not.

Those programs had it right. Small-scale farmers need financial help. Many good ideas to improve farming simply cannot be implemented by small-scale farmers due to their limited access to financing and other resources. Banks just don't like to fund risky ventures, and small operations are themselves less able to take on debt than big farms with more capital investments and larger cash flow.

But standard cost/benefit calculations may sometimes undervalue benefits—for one, sustainability is a very positive benefit. Certainly, there is a place for creative approaches as well—as with the Staps of Twin Brook Creamery, who brought in neighbors and community members to finance their glass bottling operation.

There are so many ways for government policies to support resilience. It should not be difficult, for example, to design a "resilience" requirement for participation in farm commodity programs. Participants now should comply with conservation and wetland standards; why not sign up for resilience, as well? Resilience-building steps to reduce vulnerability or risk could be more formalized in farm plans; county or regional farm services agencies could assist. Farmers could be required to show ways in which they are reducing specific risks from rising climatic temperatures, flooding streams, and resistant pests.

Here are some examples. Where there are threats from urban sprawl and resulting high land rents and nuisance ordinances, resilience planning might include taking advantage of markets and higher-valued crops sought by new neighboring residents. Threats from flooding could prompt farmers to consider a change in land use from cropping to extensive grazing or certain permaculture practices. Threats related to large, centralized sources of inputs (herbicide-laden dairy manure for organic farms, or large-scale, improperly stored forage) could be addressed by diversifying sources and types of inputs. Threats involving high energy use and extreme price spikes could prompt farmers to make a more concerted effort in on-site energy production and more self-sufficiency through energy conservation.

Although US agricultural policy calls for a "resilient," "sustainable," and "stable" system, policymakers' concept of what this entails seems to include perpetuation of an industrial model of agriculture, and it inevitably responds to vested commercial and political interests. The bias toward stability in agricultural policy and programs reflects an outdated understanding of how to achieve a system that can persist. More than ever, we live in a dynamic world of environmental, economic, and social changes and constraints that are constantly at odds with each other. Policy needs to change accordingly—to promote adaptive change and resilience.

We Need: Sustainable Fish

The situation of fish and fishing underscores even more the idea of "connections"—everything is linked together—and emphasizes the lesson that simple answers are hard to find for why foods aren't whole. A single article—"Historical Overfishing and the Recent Collapse of Coastal Ecosystems," used while I was teaching at Northwest Indian College, alerted me to problems with world fisheries—crashes in many fish populations became obvious when one looked at historic numbers. Most striking to me was that numbers of large consumer species of fish were historically "fantastically large"—there were a lot of them. And here's the clincher: particularly concerning is that decades to centuries passed from the time when overfishing occurred to when the resultant crash in numbers could be seen.

The article is wonderful storytelling and invokes many literary as well as scientific sources to uncover the evidence for such large historic numbers. It is a terrific example of interdisciplinary research—getting information from all kinds of places to find one thing. Of course, it is not without considerable controversy; the article has been cited by close to 6,000 supporters *and* critics, and in my academic world, that is a lot!

What's happening to fisheries today is startling. Fish and seafood, in all their variety, may be the world's second most important food protein source after cereal grains, accounting for about 17% of the world's protein intake (as of 2015, and increasing). Fish is generally considered good food—high in protein and high in fats. Fish consumption is increasing worldwide, and in the past few years the numbers of farmed fish—meaning, from aquaculture—have surpassed wild-caught fish. That's partly because aquaculture has been increasing, and partly because many wild stocks of fish are being steadily overharvested and are in decline.

Ocean fishing—which might be considered one of the last remnants of humankind's ancestral hunter-gatherer economy—presents a classic natural resource management dilemma, compounded by the vast distances over which many fish populations range. The resource—fish—is spread across many political jurisdictions. Fish may spend parts of their lives in streams or near-shore waters of some nations, but then other stages of their lives in the waters of other nations or the ocean far beyond any nation's boundaries. Fishing anywhere affects the populations of those fish everywhere else, and is beyond the capability of individual nations to control. Without control, everyone's incentive to harvest more fish is greater than to conserve for future years, because the benefit of catching more fish now is solely theirs while the benefit of conserving (i.e., fish not caught thus boosting future populations) is shared with all the others who may catch those fish in the future. This is a classic case of what ecologist Garrett Hardin termed the "Tragedy of the Commons" in a 1968 essay.

In the face of numerous startling cases of fish population crashes from overfishing—for example, cod on the Grand Banks off Newfoundland, bluefin tuna in the Atlantic and Mediterranean, Pacific salmon—a wide variety of national and multinational management efforts have been developed.

As we look more closely and communicate better around the globe, more instances of overfishing keep emerging. As I write this, the British newspaper *The Guardian* has just published a report on the dramatic decline—in both total weight of catch and size of individual fish—of the fish harvest off Dar es Salaam, Tanzania, East Africa, in "some of the world's richest fishing grounds" in the Indian Ocean. This is attributed to practices such as "blast fishing" with explosives, and illegal fishing including by large indiscriminate foreign trawlers.

A few weeks later the BBC, both online and on the air had reported much the same set of problems with fishing off Senegal on the west coast of Africa in the eastern Atlantic. There the problems are even more complicated, with burgeoning fish meal factories grinding vast quantities of fish into animal feed, mainly for Asia, and clashes over fish harvests with authorities in neighboring Mauritania. Everywhere we look, it seems, the story is the same.

Sustainability is generally considered the objective for fisheries management. This means harvesting the right number of the right size of fish at the right time and place so that the population can maintain itself or grow. It also means managing the other factors that affect a fish population, which all can be considered under the umbrella of "habitat." Overfishing is a huge problem, but the importance of these other factors can be seen in the example of Pacific salmon.

The five species of Pacific salmon are each a little different, but they share what is perhaps their most important characteristic: they are anadromous. That means that they spawn (i.e., reproduce) in freshwater (mainly streams), migrate far out into the ocean to grow and mature, and migrate back to freshwater to produce the next generation.

Populations of Pacific salmon are a shadow of what they once were along most of the US and Canadian coasts (populations in Alaska generally are in better shape). Often, four broad categories of causes have been blamed—the "four Hs": Harvest, Habitat, Hatcheries, and Hydroelectricity. Each "H" plays on a vulnerability somewhere in the anadromous life cycle.

Harvest as a problem is self-evident: too many fish were being caught to allow enough of them to swim upriver to spawn and produce the next generation. Habitat, in this context, is understood to mean the condition of the spawning streams (or lakes, in the case of sockeye or red salmon), the lakes or rivers or estuaries where the salmon are reared, and the oceans where the salmon grow and mature. Everything from water overuse for agriculture to contamination from urban industry damages habitat. Hatcheries—which raise Pacific salmon species from eggs and release them into the wild—seemed like such a good idea, a way to increase salmon populations for greater harvest. But in recent decades the logic of hatcheries has been challenged because of concerns about hatchery fish competing with wild populations, and concerns that the resources going into hatchery research and development might divert attention and funding from efforts to recover natural populations.

The last "H"—hydroelectricity—refers to dams. Many salmon rivers have been dammed, mostly for electric power generation, although some also provide water for irrigation and extend the range of boat transportation. Dams block salmon migration—both the adults going upstream to spawn and the young salmon coming downriver to the sea—unless accommodations are made. Many but not all dams have fish ladders, intended to allow the adults to get upriver, and some dams are managed with structures and/or procedures to help the young salmon get downriver—such as catching them and carrying them around the dams. Despite these measures, dams impede salmon. Not surprisingly, what to do about dams is highly controversial.

Aquaculture is a problematic answer to wild stock questions and issues, by FoodWISE standards. Some of the problems of aquaculture are like the problems of other kinds of livestock farming:

What are the fish fed? Often other fish, depleting the ocean biomass further and competing with wild fish for food.

Is where they're raised polluted and therefore the fish (or shellfish) contaminated? Certainly some aquaculture around the world is well managed, but artificial ponds where fish and shellfish are raised can be susceptible to pollution from runoff, and the fish food may not be well regulated.

Are the fish dosed up with hormones and antibiotics? Often, yes.

In addition, a lot of aquaculture has ecological problems not shared by most other livestock operations. A lot of fin-fish farming, particularly for Atlantic salmon, is in pens in the ocean in coastal Europe, South America, Canada, and a bit of the United States. These pens are controversial because of evidence that parasites, chemicals, and wastes from them are harmful to native wild salmon that use nearby waters. Also, Atlantic salmon sometimes escape from the pens, raising the threat of establishing populations or even interbreeding with local Pacific salmon.

Raising salmon in onshore tanks would seem to be the solution, and in fact this form of aquaculture is in the early stages of development. The standard problems of livestock farming would have to be properly managed: a sustainable food source, disease and parasite management, waste disposal, and so on. But at least the ecological impacts on wild salmon would be lessened and the genetic threats avoided.

Certainly the world wants and needs to eat fish, but ocean fishing needs to be sustainable, and farmed fish need to be healthy to eat and farmed without creating ecological problems. In particular, eating Pacific salmon in North America is FoodWISE. It's an excellent food and as unadulterated as possible, and the fishing itself is intensively managed. The five species have multiple names: what you'll see in the store are labels saying king or chinook, red or sockeye, silver or coho, chum or keta, pink or humpback. Sometimes it's just called wild salmon—then, ask what kind, and find the kind you like best for taste and affordability.

We Need: Food Security

The ideas we are discussing to put the FoodWISE philosophy into practice mostly relate to individual actions that we can take: what can we do to grow, buy, or make better food for ourselves, and what can we do to support food production systems that give us better food? Our answer to these questions has consistently been: know your source; be informed.

For many in our society, however, getting better food is a secondary problem. Getting *enough* food is the primary problem. We can't talk about food and agriculture without acknowledging the severe inequities that exist in our society in who has food. Food is about more than taste or even nutrition; it's also about who can afford it; who has access to it; and who has the time, energy, and facilities to prepare it. We need to talk about food in terms of economic strata, race, even gender identity, and the systematic marginalization of many people in our country. Ensuring food security for all is part of what we need to work toward to achieve a FoodWISE society.

Food security is having sufficient food "for an active, healthy life," by the USDA definition. It should mean not only enough calories—enough energy—from the food, but also enough of the varied nutrients we need. Furthermore, the calories that we get should come from food that nourishes— food that is high in fat and protein and fibrous carbs, and doesn't leave us only temporarily invigorated (as sugary foods do, which I discuss in Part 2).

Ensuring food security means combating food *insecurity:* not having enough food. How bad a problem is food insecurity? A lot worse than you might think.

The best information on the extent of food insecurity in the United States comes from the USDA's Economic Research Service. The ERS data are meant to guide federal government food policy and programs, which ultimately provide nutrition assistance to needy households. Numerous other information sources also track and analyze the problem, including blogs on hunger— for example, by the Food Research and Action Center (http://frac.org/blog /hunger-america-look-like) and Feeding America (www.feedingamerica.org /hunger-blog), and in reports by non-governmental organizations.

According to the ERS, close to 12% of US households lacked enough food sometime in 2017 (the most recent data available at the time of this writing).

That's 15 million households and 40 million people nationwide lacking food at least sometime during the year. If you look only at households with children under eighteen, it's almost 16% of US households. Although rates of food insecurity have been declining in the past few years, they're still higher than pre-recession (2007) levels, and 60% higher than in the 1990s, when the current method of data collection was started.

Society has mobilized a number of responses to food insecurity, with varying success. At the federal government level, we have what is intended to be a safety net in the form of nutrition assistance programs. These include the Supplemental Nutrition Assistance Program, or SNAP (formerly the Food Stamp Program), the National School Lunch Program, and the Special Supplemental Nutrition Program for Women, Infants, and Children, or WIC. The largest of these programs is SNAP; it reportedly helped more than 40 million low-income people every month in 2017 afford a nutritionally adequate diet. The National School Lunch Program provided free or reduced-price lunches to 30 million low-income students each day, and the WIC program served 7.3 million participants per month.

So, how effective are these federal nutrition assistance programs? The answer is a bit complicated. While they do provide important assistance to many millions, food insecurity still persists across the nation. About 50% of households receiving SNAP benefits were food insecure in 2017, as were 42% of households benefiting from the National School Lunch Program, and 38% of WIC benefit recipients. Clearly, participation does not guarantee that beneficiaries are free from hunger; participation does not equate to food security. Furthermore, a large percentage of households identified as "food insecure" had not participated in one or more of the government's big food assistance programs.

Many food-insecure households turn to food banks, sometimes in addition to federal assistance programs. Food banks, established by local or state governments, or sometimes nonprofit organizations, are found in many towns. Food banks collect food donations from industry, retailers, and others, including individuals; store the food; and eventually distribute it mainly to facilities like food pantries, shelters, and "soup kitchens" that in turn distribute it to individuals.

Some of this food comes from the federal government, some comes from huge retailers. Washington state, for example, has a highly centralized network of food assistance primarily relying on federal aid programs. Each month, food banks in Washington state receive over 554 truckloads of USDA food and distribute it to over 126,000 families. USDA food, trucked directly to food banks, accounts for nearly a fifth of the food that pantries distribute. The majority of the remaining food is purchased or donated from retail outlets that also get food from out of state and out of the country. Certainly, privately-run programs, at least 50,000 by some accounts, are increasing across the country, in step with increasing food needs.

Food banks pull in food from many different sources. Organizations like Feeding America (formerly called Second Harvest, the national organization for food banks) talk a lot about "rescuing" food that would otherwise be wasted to go toward feeding the hungry.

We are practically wallowing in wasted food in this country. Calories are cheap, people are picky, and policies of all sorts are counterproductive for making full use of food. From farm to table, seed to roasted vegetable, we are wasting each year almost a third (31%) of the food produced and transported in the United States. This reportedly amounts to 96 billion pounds of food and $165 billion in lost dollar value. That's a lot. Who's to blame for the food waste? Farms, grocery stores, big retailers, cafeterias, cafés, hospitals—and us. That's us cooks, a little too aggressive in chopping off what we think are the "bad parts" of fruits and vegetables, or maybe we are confused about date labeling. "Sell by" and "best if used by" Food & Drug Administration (FDA) food guidelines can be confusing. Some of the wasted food is, in fact, garbage but most is perfectly good; tens of billions of pounds of useable food end up being thrown out every year—while hunger persists.

Something better should be done with all this food, and a lot does end up in food banks. Maybe it just has a little imperfection, or maybe there's just too much produce to begin with, or too much to transport, or too much to put into cold storage, or new inventory comes in and the stock on the shelves has to go. It's not worth it to the business to salvage the older food. But, why not have it go to the food banks?

Numerous efforts to reduce waste are underway, particularly at state and local government levels and in some private food companies. Clever people are organizing social media guides to dumpster diving to extract decent food for their own use. Certainly making fuller use of the food we have is something to work on.

What else might be done to combat food insecurity? Well, a lot of places where food insecurity is concentrated—both in urban and in rural areas—are often called "food deserts." These are defined simply on the basis of access to retail food stores. The USDA's ERS defines a "low-access community," or food desert, as a census tract with at least five hundred people and/or at least 33% of the population living more than one mile from a supermarket or large grocery store in an urban area, or more than ten miles in a rural area. According to the ERS, food deserts are everywhere.

That's only part of the picture, however. Bringing a food store into a neighborhood isn't going to change food insecurity for families that don't have money to buy food at the store. On the other hand, some "low-access" communities may have other sources of food available, such as communal gardens.

People in many communities have recognized that self-help projects to grow and distribute some of their own food can be long-lasting and sustainable—more FoodWISE, in our terms—and have an important role to play in providing adequate food, maybe in combination with food assistance programs for some families. It partly depends on how we diagnose the cause of the problem.

For some community activists, like Karen Washington, cofounder of Black Urban Growers in the Bronx, New York, the causes are broader and deeper and the solutions need to involve more community development. For Washington, a recipient of a James Beard Foundation Leadership Award, change in food security is going to come more from increased capital, finance, and opportunity in the community, not from a food bank. Especially when that food bank becomes a way of life rather than an emergency relief effort.

In fact, Karen Washington considers "food desert" to be a misleading term used by outsiders that avoids recognizing the complexities of communities where getting enough good food is a problem. Better, she thinks, would be to acknowledge that the overall economic and social systems in such communities can lead to what is called "food apartheid"—a term, she says, that makes us look "at the whole food system, along with race, geography, faith, and economics."

Community efforts to improve access to food, to help neighborhoods become more FoodWISE, take many forms and are found in many places—probably including close to where you live. Here are a couple of examples close to home for me in Bellingham, Washington.

Residents of the culturally diverse (with twenty-five languages and dialects spoken) Birchwood community, an older mixed neighborhood that was mostly single-family homes and is now increasingly low-rise apartments, have been actively agitating for a supermarket ever since the large chain store Albertsons closed in 2016. The closest big market is now over a mile away.

Birchwood residents are organizing themselves to establish better access to food, especially since legal barriers to using the empty store space for another supermarket have so far stymied their lobbying—an example of how institutional barriers can help create scarcity. One initiative by the Birchwood Food Desert Fighters is regular delivery of food by truck to those who qualify to use it as a food pantry. Another is organizing Food and Garden-Share networks.

Just a few miles away from Birchwood, the Lummi Nation—Lhaq'temish, People of the Sea—deals with its own food security problems. Its solution has been to develop distribution networks to improve access to food. Its Northwest Indian College runs a service program that distributes boxes of fresh locally grown fruit and vegetables through the summer and fall. The program also participates in special food gatherings, classes, and cultural exchanges. The Lummi Food Bank is open almost every day and has served up to several hundred families each week. At the same time, the Lummi Nation makes major efforts to protect its own salmon and shellfish resources, including managing its shellfish hatchery.

Another example of urban food self-sufficiency efforts is Detroit's Georgia Street Community Collective, a nineteen-lot urban farm founded by Mark Covington in his childhood neighborhood. Other community food operations exist in Baltimore, Los Angeles, San Francisco, Austin, and in many other cities.

Has it been easy to set up the urban farms found throughout the country? Often, no. In Corktown, Detroit, Brother Nature Produce farmers tried unsuccessfully to buy the single acre of land they had used for years to produce closed-loop, all-materials-recycled vegetable produce. Eventually, they had to settle on acreage about an hour away in the county.

A common problem has been finding land to farm in a city. For one thing, those who are the most needy and vulnerable often don't have much of a say in how city land is being used. Once again, existing economic and social structures obstruct access to what is needed to improve food sources.

The Vulnerable

There is no question that many in our society are more vulnerable to food insecurity, and therefore face more challenges in living by FoodWISE principles, than others. Households identified by the USDA's ERS as vulnerable include those that are low income, those headed by a single person with children, those headed by a Hispanic or African American, and those that consist of individuals living alone. The ERS also finds geographic differences, from a low rate for food-insecure households of 7.4% in Hawaii to a high of 17.9% in New Mexico. Food insecurity rates are also higher in big cities and rural areas. These findings show, again, that existing safety nets to provide adequate food don't fully work—and that some people in some places are more affected than others. Further, there are clear economic and racial elements in who is most vulnerable.

We must put responsibility for poor participation in assistance programs, and for unemployment and underemployment, squarely in the hands of government, as well as policymakers and administrators. We need to make it easier, not harder, to access government assistance and benefits. Adding more bureaucracy to already impenetrable processes faced by the "undeserving" is not going to reduce food insecurity. Much of the interminable debates about changing government nutrition assistance programs seem to be about cutting benefits and raising bureaucratic barriers based on misguided attitudes as to why people are hungry, in effect, blaming the victims themselves.

There's something wrong with both the efficiency and the equitability of our agricultural web when we have such a big and persistent food security problem nationwide. A significant portion of our population cannot make FoodWISE decisions about their own food—it's too inaccessible and expensive.

Ironically, widespread food insecurity persists despite a considerable investment intended to alleviate the problem—for example, in fiscal year 2017, the federal government spent about $70 billion on food assistance programs.

More came from private contributions. Meanwhile, as we've seen, a lot of food is wasted or, at best, some finds its way to food supplement programs.

I'm writing this book, as I've said many times, to help readers' decision-making about food, to encourage you to learn about and take control of all aspects of your own food. But it would be irresponsible and indeed immoral not to acknowledge that this is all from a position of privilege—a position where I have the ability to make choices. Many people don't, particularly some of the most vulnerable.

We all should have the ability to make FoodWISE choices in our lives. As we learn about how the agricultural web works so that we can make better personal and communal decisions about food, so too should we push for changes that make it easier for everyone to make such choices. Food insecurity is a problem for which we all should take responsibility.

We Need: To Be FoodWISE and Choose Whole, Sustainable

I come back to the basic point that FoodWISE is essentially an approach to the many decisions we continually make around food. It offers a set of principles to help guide us, principles to follow conscientiously but flexibly—so as to be adaptive and resilient. For me, this is part of a deeply felt belief that we all need to do the right thing by each other, and seek a better future for our shared world.

The key question for our FoodWISE interests is: can the practices of large-scale as well as small-scale farms and companies also push forward broader sustainability and social justice goals? Food is not just nutrition, but also a force for achieving equity and social justice, as well as environmental protection. But it must be affordable.

Shouldn't living FoodWISE be everybody's right? Why shouldn't every person have access to food that tastes good and doesn't hurt the land? Once again, it comes back to that agricultural web: everyone is affected by food—where the food is produced, who produces it, how it is raised.

***

In Part 1, we've looked at how food affects the wider world, and how our agricultural economy could shift in directions that are more sustainable, wholesome, and resilient.

What we haven't talked much about, though, is food's effect on our own personal worlds—specifically, what food does to our bodies. How do we feed ourselves in ways that will sustain us, in a culture glutted with additives and processed foods? Why is it worth the time, effort, and expense to follow a more whole food diet, when so many cheap, processed snacks—even organic ones—fill supermarket shelves? Maybe you can already answer these questions for yourself. Still, even with the ability to pay, we don't always make the food choices we know we should. The reasons for this I will discuss in the next section.

A better world can start in the kitchen. To get to that world, though, we have to change the ways we think about food. In Part 2, we'll look at food beliefs—why we eat what we do, and why dietary changes are often so hard to make. We'll look at diets, and the science behind eating. Hopefully, by the end of the book, you'll have the tools you need on your own FoodWISE journey, figuring out what you need and what's important to you.

PART 2

Our Personal World of Food: Choosing Whole and Informed

We've been saying that FoodWISE is about making Whole-food and Whole-farm choices. Do we know where our food comes from, what's in it, how it is made? We need to be choosing delicious and whole foods within sustainable farming systems. Clearly, what we eat determines what impact we have on our planet and our communities. But what about the impact our food choices have on us, as individuals?

In the first section of Part 2, "Fierce Food Beliefs," we'll ask questions about the pervasive influence of our own food beliefs, and of advertising, on the food choices we make. This is to better understand why we make the choices we do and, if we think we need to, how to change them.

Sound information should be a major factor in making choices, and in the second section of Part 2, "Food Choices—The Informed Science of Eating," we'll take a tour through science. How can we use science to better inform ourselves about food? What do different foods actually do in our bodies? How do we retrain ourselves to recognize the foods that are good for us, and what does "good for us" even mean? Part 2 is not meant to be an exhaustive nutritional survey of specific foods and their function in our bodies. Nor is the "Fierce Food Beliefs" section meant to demonize advertising for influencing our food choices—but advertising is nonetheless an important factor. Another issue is the lack of choice in whole foods, which leaves us with sugary manufactured foods. Aided and abetted by formidable advertising, as well as by our own food beliefs, we often don't think about our food choices. The purpose of Part 2, then, is to offer some information on how and why we make the food choices we do, and nudge us in a more FoodWISE direction.

SECTION 1: FIERCE FOOD BELIEFS

Are there foods you know you should be eating and foods you know are bad for you? Do some dishes seem to have a remarkable ability to heal you when you're sad or sick? Could that healing be just a placebo effect, and does that matter, if it works?

We also want to know how particular patterns of eating affect satiety, or how full we feel, or change our sense of well-being. Does a big breakfast make a difference in how hungry you feel a few hours later, can you really eat a little buckwheat and be happy for the day? If you ditch the sugar, will you really stop thinking about it? The common question underlying all these others is: How can we separate our food beliefs and attitudes from "hard facts," and is there value in overruling facts with feelings some of the time?

Without the process of scientific inquiry, it is difficult to make informed choices about our food. But science won't have all the answers: our own feelings, our priorities, and the yearnings of our own palates are factors only we ourselves can roll into our decision-making. There's interesting scientific information that can inform us on many questions. But sometimes we can't see or hear it, because our fierce food beliefs get in the way. Let's look at how these beliefs affect us, and where they come from. Since our beliefs, grounded in reality or not, inspire our action, along the way we'll look at the diet culture in America, driven by our beliefs about food.

So, let's begin with this: Part of being FoodWISE is trusting our own instincts. Every decision in the garden, the grocery store, or the kitchen is colored by the entire history of our relationship with food. Where does that relationship come from, and how can we take apart and recognize the influences of our parents, mass media, and our own research as we make those decisions?

My mother had many food beliefs, and I must admit they have rubbed off on me. Milk was important—she told me it would help build strong bones. Every day before going off to school she made sure I had two nickels wrapped in a handkerchief and tied off with a rubber band. My mother tucked the coins in my pocket, and I would use them to buy a small carton of milk. She also had some pretty magical beliefs about "brain food": eat liver or fish (or that milk I bought) and you will grow smarter. Fortunately, she limited lunch fare to sandwiches made from canned fish (more like what my classmates were eating), saving liver for dinner.

Is my brain better because of this? I'd like to think so. Fish do contain key omega-3 fatty acids, though I'm not sure my mother knew this when I was growing up. And that's the thing: many of us hold strong food beliefs that have nothing to do with science or accepted fact. Anything—from childhood associations to the power of advertising—can affect what we believe about food. And those beliefs wind up shaping our food choices.

Beliefs help us organize the world and make it more controllable. We fear what we don't understand. We form beliefs in order to clarify and interpret information or situations we observe. We like to know the future! *I expect this food to taste this way, it will have this effect on my body and my mood, I'll make it just the way my mother did, and everything will be all right.* What happens, though, when different people hold different beliefs— when a Safeway ad tells us that our mother's clam chowder isn't as good as theirs, or when we learn from our friend who's a biologist that seafood contains mercury?

We live in an age of information overload, and the steady stream of information we get from friends, scientists, TV, the internet, and countless other sources influences our beliefs, opinions, and habits. With so many opinions to choose from, beliefs, instead of guiding us, sometimes start to get in our way. Whom to believe? Why? And how do we get past that intuition that a food we're told is unhealthy might be exactly what we need?

Our beliefs also can evolve as we gain new information. We just need to recognize how old beliefs have formed, and develop ways to pick up new information—including ways to decide what new information is sound. Family lore and traditions, gut feelings, personal experience, social networks, advertising, news in the media, and actual scientific findings all come into it.

Many of us rely on our gut feelings: *My family used to make this, it must be good,* or, *This has fat, I don't want to get fat; therefore I'd better not eat it.* Sometimes we don't even know where our beliefs about food come from. One of the first steps to becoming FoodWISE is to get to the bottom of our beliefs: why do we feel the way we do about food, and does it make sense? How, say, would we consider chocolate if we didn't already have beliefs about and associations with it? If we want to change how we eat—if we want to become FoodWISE eaters—it makes sense to start by thinking about *how* we think about food.

The Raisin That Wasn't

Clearly, ideas we have about food influence our eating behavior. We're surrounded by contradictory messages about what we should eat, how much, and when. Experience, association, and memory tell us so much about what we "should" eat that it's hard to listen to our stomachs or our rational minds. Food is *never* "just food." It's food with associations. This means that the same food can be experienced by two different people in entirely different ways.

Food beliefs may be deep-seated in their complicated origins, and stubborn, but personal experience can change perceptions and help start changing beliefs. New sensory experiences with food—especially taste but also sight and even sound (the crunch of crisp celery!)—can modify the positive (or negative) associations with different foods that we may have developed as early as childhood. Sometimes we make those associations in surprising ways.

Years ago our then–twenty-month-old son was cooking side-by-side with his twin sister and stirring a thick batter with chocolate chips, supervised by my friend Teresa while I went out to do errands. Teresa, seeing the look on my face, said, "Don't worry, he won't eat them." But, sure enough, when I returned home I heard that he'd eaten a chip that had fallen out of the bowl—his first taste of chocolate. *Alas,* I thought, (this, I realize now, was an expression of my own food beliefs) *the slippery slope to self-indulgent eating, an obsession with chocolate, a life of unmitigated snacking on sweets.* However, my son merely reported: "That was a *really* good raisin."

To me, chocolate is an emotion-laden food. It's *chocolate:* the ultimate gastronomic vice (or delight)! Not in my son's world, though. He had no associations: chocolate wasn't yet romance or indulgence, heart attack or reward. My son, like every eater everywhere, expected one experience and got another: for him, that food now *was* a "raisin," never mind that it didn't taste or look quite like any raisin he had had before. The actual experience of eating this "raisin" was different than everything he already thought he knew about what he was eating; his perceptions changed his belief about raisins. And from that, they changed his choices; for sure, from then on he was on the lookout for the good raisins.

Maybe our son didn't notice the slightly different shape and texture of the "raisin"; maybe he did and was game to experiment. If so, then something he didn't have was *neophobia,* being fearful of trying new things. In the process of trying new foods, he was building associations, part of a memory strategy. For those neophobes among us it's simple: no new foods, no new memories. But we can't spend our entire lives sustained by childhood foods, right? Instead, let's embrace a bigger consciousness about food.

Food Choices: Experience, Quality, and Beliefs

Good reasons exist for caution in choosing foods. Foods that don't taste like those of our gastronomic histories—too bitter, too spicy, too moldy—could be dangerous. Sometimes, though, those cautions prevent us from trying good foods we've never tasted. We might choose a lower-quality (less Whole) mass-produced white bread on the grocery store shelf, say, simply because it's all we've ever been exposed to, and a bland taste and soft texture have become our norm. This is how beliefs get between us and our plates: we don't look for good-tasting alternatives because we believe we already know which foods we like the most.

My favorite example is olive oil. If we have never tasted an early-season olive oil, one that "burns" the throat, then we might accept as satisfactory any oil labeled, say, "extra virgin." In blind tasting exercises at the University of Florence, my students, and the Italian students too, chose rancid sunflower seed oil as their "olive oil" of choice. This bland, non-pungent vegetable oil was a low-quality oil that in no way met Italian and international standards for acidity that would apply to a fine olive oil. The students, though, preferred its taste, believing it was the best oil; it fit with their previous perceptions and experiences of "olive oil," since much of what's sold in the United States is a cheaper, milder oil. I suppose it's not surprising that we choose the familiar. But, particularly with olive oils, we're losing the more interesting, high nutrient ones, with phenolic compounds that give extra virgin olive oil a bitter, spicy flavor and maybe a hefty antioxidant load.

Okay—but does it matter? If we're happy with the cheap substitute, who cares if we never know the difference? Well, those blander, rancid oils might work in a salad, but they certainly won't benefit a rich tomato sauce, one that calls for an oil that you can feel in the back of your throat even as the tomatoes seductively sweeten the effect. In the case of oils, we're losing out on nutrients as well as taste. For one thing, fresh oil contains a lot of valuable compounds that old oil doesn't. For another, what happens when we eat that inferior tomato sauce? We may not know exactly what's wrong with it, but we will know it's not satisfying—so we add some more salt/cheese/sugar/ artificial something to that pasta, further drowning the delicate purity of one simple dish.

I'm all for the affordable price of store-brand olive oil, but let's also have the quality. Quality for me is about flavor, smells, textures of whole food dishes. Adequate access to food should imply access to high-quality food, especially if the price point is acceptable. ("Price point" is a handy marketing term for the intersection of price and quality considerations—a perfect concept for our study of food.) But that's just it—how do you balance price with quality? This is a key question asked by food sensory scientists. We'll be looking at their ideas about the importance of food quality later on.

As we've seen with olive oil, though, even "quality" itself is hard to determine. If we're told enough times that a food is "good," we start to believe it, and the memory of real good food—that early-season olive oil, for example—fades away into oblivion or never was on our radar to begin with. Is "cheap" good? Is rancid good? Corporations concerned with profit are quick to answer "yes—just buy it." The tool they use to convince us to make that choice is advertising.

Advertising: We Eat What We're Told

We know that our sustainable, resilient, equitable agricultural web is strengthened—nationally and locally—when we make whole food choices. These include choices away from processed foods—heavy in corn and soy, typically produced on mono- or duo-crop farms with little farm-generated fertility. I think it's fairly accurate to say that our big-brand barbeque chips aren't coming from integrated farms. So, do we choose organic chips? How do we decide? What are the influences on our decisions? It is clear that beliefs drive our choices, and in our very connected world, advertising has become a major influence on shaping our beliefs.

Advertising presents information—words, pictures, sounds, colors—to persuade us to buy a particular product or service. The labels on food products can be considered another front in the persuasion battle waged by companies to win us over, as much as a medium of useful information. Labels on food packages influence consumers in various ways. "Low-fat" labels strongly influence food buying, even when the calorie content is not much different than that of other foods. Tags such as "new," "improved," and "healthy" also sell products, regardless of how new or improved they actually are. Even wine labels have considerable influence. Did you know that the place name (a California chardonnay vs. a South Carolina one) can affect how much wine you drink, which in turn affects how much food you consume? A homey label helps—like "Grandma's" sugar cookies. Everyone knows that fat is bad, right? And homemade is better? Advertisers play on beliefs like these, giving consumers as many reasons as possible to think that buying this food, now, is the best choice they have.

Advertising is persuasive—especially if it has some science to back it up—and aims to be successful at building customer loyalty. You can't sell completely crummy food, at least not for long. But don't underestimate the ability to sell foods by invoking a bit of science in the advertising to make the product seem more reputable.

It's trite but true that advertising is everywhere: on the web, in the news-paper, in magazines, on TV. Of course, how much we encounter depends on how many of these outlets we frequent and how often. Children are partic-ularly susceptible to advertising, and perhaps older teens as well, especially when they're also keyed into the advertising-fueled idea of material posses-sions as necessary for happiness and success. For all of us, a bit of a story or a little humor and music go a long way. When we're shown the people we *want* to be, of course we're going to try to imitate. We form beliefs about foods, and at the same time we're forming beliefs about ourselves.

One prime example: coffee.

The growth of specialty or gourmet coffees and the prices consumers pay are a continuing trend in many parts of the world—for instance, almost 60% of coffee was consumed outside the home in the United States in 2017: more people drinking specialized coffee, and drinking more cups per day. Coffee—grown and produced in Latin America, Asia, East Africa, and elsewhere—once was available for pennies to consumers in developed countries. Now, though, it costs quite a few pennies to get an espresso. Has this hike in price made coffee consumption go down? Not at all. Coffee has become such a cultural necessity that many of us hand over our dollars to Starbucks on a daily basis without a second thought. It isn't even just about the taste. Starbucks tastes good, don't get me wrong.

For many of us, though, our very self-image is tied up to that cup of joe. How many of us describe ourselves as "coffee people"? Don't we go on "coffee dates" to get out of the house, or measure our pride in getting through a work deadline by how many cups of coffee fueled us on the way? Coffee shows you work hard. Coffee shows you have class: not everyone can afford Starbucks, after all. Tastes change—now this latte is in style, now we like dark roasts, now we like light. What doesn't change is the role our consumption plays in our identity, our conceptions and constructions of ourselves: "I'm a coffee drinker." It's how we know ourselves. The coffee may be tasty, but the interlocking influence of advertising and culture helps form these ideas of what coffee means to us. And maybe we like the "cultural crusader" part of Starbucks's messaging, too.

Wait: this isn't reasonable. My identity is tied up with the fact that I drink a particular beverage? Well, it's looking that way. And other examples make even less sense. Take tap water. Even in the United States, where tap water is generally safe (chlorination-fluoridation issues notwithstanding), we consume billions of bottles of packaged water each year. We've made bottled water our number one beverage, spending $18.5 billion on 13.7 billion gallons in 2017—over 42 gallons per person.

All the plastic in these bottles creates a serious environmental waste problem, not to mention the energy consumed in manufacture and transport. With water, advertising has managed to take a (mostly) readily available, free resource and turn it into a designer item, convincing consumers that it tastes better, is better for us … and we're better people for drinking it. Say farewell to municipally monitored tap water, say hello to expensive plastic bottles of pretty much the same stuff. In fact, much bottled water is actually from a tap. But we congratulate ourselves when we buy a bottle of water at the concession stand: hey, we're not buying soda pop. Just like with coffee, there's a certain identity we think we acquire by being bottled-water drinkers.

As we go through our day, we can see many other examples of advertising shaping our beliefs about ourselves and our beliefs about food. Advertising's job is to produce positive associations between things we already feel good about and things to buy. Those labels I mentioned earlier? Picture that wine label showing a beautiful hillside vineyard or a cookie package with a loving grandma in an old-fashioned kitchen. Such images evoke positive, pleasurable feelings—basically, happiness we can buy (we'll talk about this a bit more later).

It's worth noting that advertising succeeds when it raises this happiness motivation above the other values we hold in making food choices. What about environmental sustainability—the impacts of plastic bottles? What about social and cultural equity—the living and working conditions of coffee farmers? What about whole foods—the ingredients in those "old-fashioned" cookies?

Selling Time: Convenience and Advertising

Many foods these days, from drive-through coffee to vending-machine bottled water and chips, have another strong appeal: convenience. Even if we're not out to buy happiness, we may be convinced to buy time. Advertising promises convenience, and that might get even the more reluctant among us to the supermarket shelves.

It wasn't very long ago that people (mostly women) whipped up dinners from scratch and knew exactly what went into each dish; if they lived outside cities, they might have picked it from the garden that morning. Most of their decisions about what to eat were made long before they got into the kitchen. Food advertising existed, but the available choices were so much more limited that personal decisions and planning carried more weight, and took considerably more time and effort.

Today, most of us make these decisions at the last minute, practicing Constant Convenience Consumerism, a phrase I borrowed from author Sandor Katz. What are we going to pick up on the way home to feed the family? What did we stock our shelves with months ago that we can eat today? Often, the biggest factor in our choices is convenience. Is it easy? Can I find a drive-through? Will my kids be happy that I bring "the take out" home so we can have a pleasant dinner? If "yes," then full steam ahead.

Convenience counts for a lot. The longer shelf life of processed foods means they're in the pantry when we want them, and fewer pennies are wasted on spoiled food. Processed foods, or more broadly "convenience foods," include breakfast cereals, sugary drinks, Cheetos, Twinkies, pastries—all these foods translate into a lot of calories that can be eaten in a short amount of time, and don't require much effort to prepare or store.

However, notice that none of these foods are whole foods. Most convenience foods have undergone a great deal of transformation, from the original whole food state of their ingredients (think milk, nuts, wheat, sugarcane) to the vegetable-oil-sugar-flour-plus-preservatives mix that winds up in packages at the store. Such processed foods raise questions. Are these no longer whole fats and sugars our bodies can use? Or, are we getting fructose without the fiber, or processed fats our bodies can't utilize?

Don't get me wrong here. Convenience does matter. Anything short of slaughtering your own chickens is a boon to overworked housewives, and we're well past the age when a woman's place (or anyone's place) should be in the kitchen. Today, much of home consumption centers on prepared foods. A nationwide survey of grocery purchases found that, "More than 80 percent of calories were purchased in ready-to-eat or ready-to-heat form in 2012, and these tended to be higher in fat, sugar and salt than food purchases that required preparation."

Sales of convenience foods such as prepared meals, meal replacement bars, and frozen food (from raw vegetables to whole meals) are particularly important to families with one parent or with both parents working. We need the time convenience foods give us. For many households, food security is now defined not by a pantry full of raw ingredients, but by the availability of nearby prepared food, whether that food is handed to them through a drive-through window, in a take-out order, or a packaged meal purchased at a grocery store.

For large food corporations, this is good news. Foods that are chock-full of preservatives, additives, and chemicals have a great shelf life and turn a great profit. Better yet, their added ingredients lend themselves well to advertising. "Fortified" grains, for example, may have had a lot added to them—after their original goodness had been stripped out. And it doesn't take much to create a product you can advertise as "reduced sugar" or "less fat" if the standard you're starting from is, well, Twinkies.

No question, convenience is important. I'm glad that I don't have to use baker's ammonia for leavening (although I still do for some holiday baking). Baking powder was an early convenience food embraced by the "modern housewife" according to *Twinkie, Deconstructed* author Steve Ettlinger, opening the door to chemical leavening and faster baking.

We talked about access to food in Part 1. Many families who don't have good access to food are desperate for a cheap, easy meal their kids will unquestioningly eat. Even if they could get whole ingredients, many can't afford the wasted food a neophobe child might refuse to eat, or the additional prep time of fresh vegetables and meats. This could apply to all of us. Such considerations sell an awful lot of frozen chicken nuggets.

Many of us, though, buy our convenience foods only because ... well, because we *think* we need them. In her book *Food Politics: How the Food Industry Influences Nutrition and Health,* food writer and activist Marion Nestle highlights the ways in which advertisers make us think we're buying foods both new and necessary when we cruise down those convenience store aisles. More recently, author Michael Ruhlman presented data on how, in less than thirty years, the country has gone from an average of 7,000 items in a grocery store to more like 40–50,000. That's a lot of products to choose from—and many of them are convenience foods. In all this vast array of foods, how many are whole, and not just another combination of corn and soy, or of sugar, processed fat, and salt?

That is journalist Michael Moss's take on food retail in his book *Salt Sugar Fat: How the Food Giants Hooked Us.* Moss focuses on the food industry and details how companies like Nestlé, Kellogg's, General Mills, and Nabisco jostle for market share. These corporations share a pervasive fear that something might happen to cut into their business—like a surgeon general leading a battle against overeating, similar to what happened with the anti-cigarette campaigns in earlier decades. Or a movement arising that would undercut their corporate response to increasing concerns about obesity ("exercise more"). If you stop—think—then act as you consider these convenience foods, don't you get a little skeptical about the advertising claims when you think about how much money is involved?

Moss also discusses new food products designed specifically to create a craving. This is a move by manufacturers to capitalize on our brains' chemical "bliss point"—a physiological reaction to certain combinations of sugar, fat, and salt that make particular foods all but irresistible. As we try to balance all our rational considerations in making our food choices, the effects of what we could call cravings (or, at the very least, persistent food thoughts) and other physiological signals only complicate our decisions.

Marion Nestle warns that any nutritional message advertisers give us is suspect, especially when it comes from for-profit industries. Yes, some food manufacturers have responded to pressure by moves like lowering sugar in cereals—but levels still remain close to Moss's "bliss point" in order to maintain sales. Nestle's point is simple: Environmental factors make it impossible to sensibly choose the foods we need to eat. By "environmental" she means the combination of social, commercial, and institutional influences on food choice that surround us—including all those things advertisers rely on to sell their products. The lure of convenience is too great.

Nestle has been at this for a while. As a food policy advocate, she has reviewed countless Federal Register notices, congressional hearing reports, acts of Congress, General Accounting Office reports, and releases of agency advisories to the food industry. Through it all, she keeps making the same discoveries: food companies know exactly what they're doing in terms of pushing the bliss-point foods. And, until something changes, the calculated allure of convenience foods high in fat, sugar, and salt will keep the American public wanting more.

Advertising Health

As we've said, advertising is all about trying to shape what we want. In its never-ending efforts to convince us to buy, it's also effective at telling us what we need (or think we need). This may be certain ingredients in food, or separate supplements to ingest such as vitamins, minerals, and protein powders. Supplements may make sense, but not because they necessarily "boost immunity" or "give energy." Advertising is selling health, but is it the health we actually need?

In our world of fortified juices and breakfast cereals, it may be hard to imagine a time when vitamins were lacking. Yet ships' logs and other writings of a few hundred years ago, from long sailing expeditions with little fresh fruit and vegetables, give some perspective on what became known as scurvy:

> A dread disease its rankling horror shed,
>
> And death's dire ravage through mine army spread.
>
> Never mind eyes such dreary sight beheld,
>
> Ghastly the mouth and gums enormous swell'd...

In fact, the experiment in the mid-1700s by Scottish physician James Lind showing that citrus fruit (which contains vitamin C) prevents scurvy was one of the earliest connections made scientifically between a food and a disease. Other cultural medical histories go back even farther. Rickets (vitamin D deficiency) and scurvy have been documented since Greek and Roman times, and reportedly the Chinese knew how to prevent it on long sea voyages as early as the 1400s. Anemia can be traced from the Neolithic era through to the Bronze Age, and later. Notably, most hunter-gatherer cultures don't seem to have had too many micronutrient deficiencies, indicating a more varied diet with a better intake of protein.

How do these historical discoveries affect our eating patterns now? Purported diet solutions to historical medical issues have become prime opportunities for advertising—which often moves beyond solving a particular problem and into claims of broader and more sweeping preventative abilities or health benefits. From understanding that vitamins can treat deficiency diseases, it's a short mental leap to "more is better." Food corporations help us make that leap with advertising for protein and other nutrient powders, and claims for the natural constituents or the additives in certain "whole and healthy" packaged foods. The idea that we can boost health with high consumption of a particular nutrient goes way back. None of this has been lost on food corporations. Walk down the grocery aisle and read all those bright labels: *Fortified with vitamins x and y! 100% of your daily requirement! Eight whole grains and 80 whole vitamins in every slice!*

A major influence on our shopping is the belief that we should choose the right combination of food components: vitamins and carbohydrates and fats and proteins and calories and cell-protective antioxidants. Instead of cultivating a taste for healthy and satiating foods, we begin to see food in terms of nutrients—either in excess (fats, for example) or deficit (vitamins). Journalist Michael Pollan calls this obsession with particular nutrients *nutritionism*. Pollan plaintively asks, in *In Defense of Food,* Whatever happened to *just* food? But nutritionism is something that can be promoted—aided by advertising and other marketing, especially to consumers who are short on time and money and seeking quick fixes rather than mentally draining analyses of what's the "right" food.

The obsession with nutrients sidetracks us into believing that nutrient-fortified food is good for us, despite it being loaded with sugar and other simple carbs (which break down quickly to provide energy). I must admit that when I first started teaching, I practiced my own version of this component-centered nutritionism, using a USDA Handbook to devise exercises for determining protein content of foods. I thought this was a good way to have students carefully look at the type and amount of foods they were eating. (A side benefit was that it gave us a perfect excuse to share recipes and cook a gigantic meal together.) For the record, I didn't tout "the more protein, the better."

Today we are awash in advice on what to eat and when and how. We're constantly told what's good for us and what's bad. But, as discussed earlier, what we hear is not at all consistent and much of it seems contradictory. Do protein supplements impart health, or just make for expensive urine? How can we learn what foods fulfill the same nutritional requirements, but in whole form?

I want to reiterate that learning how to evaluate sources of information, and how to benefit from the ever-expanding body of scientific information, is an important tool for our FoodWISE decision-making. Rather than learn which foods are good or bad, or whom to listen to and trust, it's better to improve our skill in being able to figure that out for ourselves. For one thing, today's best answers may change tomorrow. For another, the best answers may be different for different people.

"Diets" can be thought of as being the health advice for lots of different food items pulled together and packaged into one overall system. Let's now look at the selling of diets for health, both because advertising and promoting diets represents a major form of influence over our food choices, and to see how we can evaluate the kind of food information we are bombarded with.

Believing Diets

Diets are the epitome of belief systems. People cope with their hundreds of daily food choices by picking a particular set of foods they will (or won't) eat: a diet. So, people attempt to buy health by buying into patterns of eating that they believe will provide it for them. A "diet" strictly means the sum of all the food you eat. However, types of diets—low-carbohydrate, or low-fat, or low-calorie, or high-protein—have come to popularly mean systems of selecting or restricting particular foods.

Diets have become big business. Some diets are proprietary plans—often named after the founder—and subscribers pay for hand-holding, inspiration, and even food (often highly processed) to carry them through. Some are mostly principles; you can feed yourself according to the ideas of the "paleo" or the "Mediterranean" diet. Today we have blood-type diets, anti-aging diets, detoxification diets, cellulite-removing diets, and innumerable others. Some diets deify one food—maybe kale, grapefruit, or green smoothies—to the exclusion of others.

About 45 million Americans in the United States go on diets each year, buying into a $60-billion diet industry. Pills, supplements, and diet convenience foods are a part of this bill. And the worse that information in the media makes us feel about ourselves, the more desperate we will be to spend our money on whatever it tells us to.

At the heart of the appeal of diets are beliefs about what our bodies should be—and, particularly, look—like. Some of this is based on data: obesity is shown to be a factor in various health problems. But some is cultural, derived from that same complex of messages we receive from the world around us that shapes our other beliefs about food.

A main belief we have is an obsession with thinness. This leads us—particularly those of us who are female—to adopt dietary plans that promise body perfection. An extreme but common case is the set of widely held body ideals for female ballet dancers and runway models, which leads teenage girls to anorexia and bulimia. Disordered eating may be even stronger for female college students, with sometimes disastrous effects. Ultra-thin, ultra-fit, and ultra-sexy images are important contributors. But even for older adult women, social media, magazine covers, swimsuit ads, and TV shows all provide abundant images of what someone else thinks our female bodies should look like. (The same applies to men to a less pernicious degree, with images such as underwear models with six-pack abs.)

In truth, as we all actually know deep down, most female bodies never could look like the models in any ad, or even in Instagram feeds—carefully shot, curated, and Photoshopped. More to the point, for our FoodWISE discussion, our food choices are only partly responsible for our shape and size, anyway. There's also our genetic makeup, how intensively we exercise, whether we smoke … the list goes on. In fact, allowing our bodies to get the fuel they need and maintain the shape that's natural for each of us will get most of us a lot closer to the body we want, without dieting and without starving.

Weight is a complex topic and I don't pretend to cover it. But here are a few points worth keeping in mind.

A discussion of diets, food restriction, and weight loss needs to recognize how much we have pathologized obesity. Food writer Julie Guthman takes on what she sees as the nation's obsession with thinness and disparagement of fat in *Weighing In: Obesity, Food Justice, and the Limits of Capitalism*. She argues that state and federal agencies battle the "obesity epidemic" with missionary zeal, hoping to "civilize" the masses into focusing on low-fat (and usually high-sugar) foods. She also notes that those same agencies are responsible for a food policy that encourages the production of commodity crops (corn and soy) that are the foundation for processed and convenience foods. Guthman is squarely in the same camp as Marion Nestle and Michael Moss. No matter how many convivial meals, group potlucks, or USDA food pyramid school lunch meals are served, that still doesn't change the easy availability of so much unwholesome food: high in sugar, salt, and processed fat.

The dieting mentality is to eat less, for a limited time, to dial into your target number on a scale. Food becomes a fixation dictated by an external program, rather than a set of choices supported by awareness of physical needs and, say, sustainable food production practices. For many who use the problematic approach of food restriction, backlash and backsliding are nearly impossible to avoid. Restricting food does not mean our obsessions with it go away.

Furthermore, weight gain is not merely a question of eating too much of the "wrong foods" (i.e., fats) and/or exercising too little. Results from the Women's Health Initiative Dietary Modification Trial—a large-scale clinical trial with almost 50,000 women over eight years—certainly didn't show what was expected. It looked at weight and also cancer and cardiovascular disease. It found that a low-fat diet did not appear to reduce these.

Wait—what? Eating less fat doesn't necessarily mean we'll lose weight? That's right: we are built to adapt to adverse circumstances, and when our bodies start getting signals that not enough food is coming in, they quickly compensate. A body expending energy draws on carbohydrates first; that's why athletes will bulk up on carbs right before a big game or long race. When not enough calories are going in and not enough carb stores exist, the body uses a specific metabolic adaptation: ketosis. This process converts fat and protein fragments into what are known as ketone bodies. These ketone bodies are an alternative fuel that allows the body to continue working when carbohydrates—that go-to energy source—are lacking. In severe restriction, the body can mobilize amino acids, which degrades protein tissue in muscles and organs. This is not a good situation—but it does result in survival during severe calorie restriction. Breaking down your body tissue is not a good long-term way for your body to get the calories it needs. Soon, the body begins to need fewer calories, as fat requires relatively fewer calories to maintain itself than those now-depleted muscle stores would have required. And upon refeeding? The additional intake goes to weight gain. More importantly, the body does not forget this poor attempt to restrict calories.

And thus, the problem gets worse each time a dieter "yo-yos," losing weight and then gaining it again. Once again, it's an issue of adaptation: with each restrictive phase, fat or adipose cells respond by becoming increasingly more efficient at storing fatty acids. When we go back to dieting, our bodies remember the last time and are not amused. It's even harder to lose weight the next time around. My point is that trying to get to some idealized condition of thin by repeatedly restricting calories in this way doesn't even work.

So why does the modern diet culture continue to thrive? Largely because we cling to advertising-fueled beliefs about what we should look like and how to get there: low-fat, low-calorie, and (incidentally) high-sugar foods. But information from the National Weight Control Registry suggests that "successful" diets—those whose adherents are happy with the results of their new way of eating—almost always include making serious lifestyle as well as food changes.

Think about it. Doesn't it make sense that a lifestyle of diet-food consumerism feeds our obsession with appearance, weight, and various well-being indicators? The important thing to remember here: stop—think—then act. Think FoodWISE—Whole foods, Informed choices, Sustainable farms, tasty food Experiences. None of that is possible in a world of convenience consumerism, where whole fats are excluded and sugar is everywhere. So, let go of the blissful foods and find some more wholesome alternatives. A little provocative science is going to help show us how we can evaluate the mass of information available, come to our own conclusions, and—in the end—question some of our fierce food beliefs.

SECTION 2: FOOD CHOICES—THE INFORMED SCIENCE OF EATING

Wow—what a lot of diet strategies to think about! Eat carbs, not fat; eat fat, not carbs; go vegetarian; eat meat and a whole lot of it. Clearly some of these diets must work better than others. Clearly some of them may be totally wrong!

It's easy to get overwhelmed by all the contradictory information found in media and in dieting culture. How can we ever figure out what's "right"? Well, the first thing I'll say is that "right" is always subjective. "Right" ultimately should mean what's right for you. But there are definitive things we can say about most of these diets if we use one tool at our disposal: science. Respectable science doesn't lie. The key is to determine what "respectable" science is.

It is true we crave simple answers to our questions about diet, but the science behind the proclamations of diet pundits is rarely as simple as they would have us believe. The truth is, answers are complex, with many considerations.

We can ask simple questions, but it's not easy to get simple answers (I surely don't have them!). Yet scientific information is worth digging through to find the FoodWISE buried in there.

Science is about systematic questioning and exploration: studies should be repeatable (preferably by other researchers) and generate similar results each time, creating reliable knowledge that doesn't come from just one person in one lab. I call this respectable science. Science is not necessarily completely objective—inevitably the choices of what to study and how to frame research and interpret results are subjective—but done reputably it does aim for honesty, completeness, and transparency about goals, methods, and actual results. Is this enough? I think so.

But you can't decide how big a role science should play in your food choices until you know which claims result from respectable science, and which have no basis in science. "Everyone is entitled to his own opinion, but not to his own facts," as Daniel Patrick Moynihan memorably put it. So, I want to take a good look at science, in terms of results we already are aware of, as well as new, provocative ideas.

Every day, social media and popular websites share "new studies" purporting to upend food science dogma. Many of them are simply repackaged from one another, with few actual new discoveries, and are only sometimes based on scientifically rigorous studies. To know what scientific findings merit our consideration, it's essential to understand a little bit about how respectable science works.

Maybe you've come across the quotes below on cholesterol from an article that appeared a few years ago in the *New York Daily News* and was widely reprinted and repackaged—and paraded as scientific reporting: "Think twice before you bite into a hearty breakfast of eggs benedict slathered in hollandaise sauce—you may as well be lighting up, according to a new study," the article begins. It warns that in terms of cardiovascular disease, "the yolk-based sauce that makes the dish so good is almost as bad for you as smoking cigarettes"—this is supposedly what researchers in Canada found.

In fact, the article drew on research in Canada that found that eating cholesterol-rich egg yolks was implicated in buildups of waxy plaque in our carotid arteries (those that supply blood to our head). The article leaps past these actual findings and the research's cautiously worded conclusions to state emphatically that, first of all, eating eggs *causes* the plaque buildup (which is different than *implicated)*, and then that consuming the eggs, and presumably the controversial cholesterol in them, does as much harm to our organs by critically blocking blood flow as does smoking cigarettes.

However, other scientists emphasize that there are complex factors in heart problems and come to different conclusions about what blame can be attributed to eggs. For instance, a paper summarizing presentations at a conference in 2011 on the relationship between dietary cholesterol intake and cardiovascular disease risk noted that a number of epidemiological studies had not shown the predicted positive relationship between cholesterol intake and cardiovascular disease. That's true, too, for recent clinical trials, looking at the effects of long-term egg intake (and thus dietary cholesterol)—results suggest no negative impact on cardiovascular health and related diseases. In fact, the researchers concluded that eggs are a "healthy" food and sensible strategies are needed to include them in diets.

As consumers struggling to know what to think, what do we do with all this? First of all, we've done the right thing by looking into the topic further and finding other research results. Second, the contradiction among the studies (much less, among popular articles) is reason enough for us to at least question what effect dietary cholesterol actually has in our bodies, rather than blindly accepting either position. Then, when we look further, we find even more research results that cast doubt on the effects of eggs.

Why, then, have we been told for so long to stay away from eggs? To answer this question, we need to know what to look for in respectable research.

Understanding the organization of the research is a good place to start. Western science typically shares its story in a prescribed way. There's a statement of a hypothesis or idea or question, a review of what's been done around that question, details of the specific data collection process, and analysis and discussion of results presented in the discussion of the data. Invariably, there are recommendations for future research, and cautionary statements about study interpretation. Papers often contain disclaimers on the limits of the work, including why people shouldn't generalize from specifics of the research. These are all important elements to look for.

But generalizing beyond the legitimate scope of the findings is precisely what the popular press often does. With the egg study / cigarette comparison example, the commentators should have looked carefully at the researchers' disclaimers: while the people eating eggs in one study saw a rise in blood cholesterol, there could be a lot of other factors affecting that. The results could have to do with a lack of exercise, for example, or a partiality for Twinkies, or sleep deprivation, the stress of constant arguing with your spouse, taking prescription drugs, or basking in the light of a full moon.

While these findings about cholesterol are worth considering, we just don't know the full story unless and until someone has researched all these questions. We don't know anything about the subjects of the Canadian study except that they did indeed eat eggs, and they did indeed have unhealthy arteries. Does this constitute conclusive science? Well, I know I'd want to learn a lot more before I used this study as a reason to give up my morning egg(s). Simply put, a credible diet study needs to be as comprehensive as possible, taking into consideration many contributing factors. Even if subjects report substantial changes, it may be years before the full results of diet modifications are evident.

The last thing to consider is scientific bias. Despite our best efforts, it's impossible to conduct science without some bias creeping in. It is so easy to introduce partiality at any point along the way. Which questions are you asking, and are you hoping for one result over another? Who is paying for your research, and is there some sort of reward (if only notoriety or fame) if your results show a particular result?

One particularly nefarious example is that of the sugar industry funding research in the 1960s that downplayed the danger of sugar and blamed fat as a health hazard. A good review article on this topic talks about how industry sponsoring of research on soft drinks, juice, and milk really can affect the results of the research itself.

The researchers found that out of 111 academic articles that declared their financial sponsorship, almost none of those funded by industry showed unfavorable results for their industry's product. This bias is precisely what we must be on the lookout for as we review a study's findings and funding.

One flagrant type of bias is what's known as "cherry-picking." Cherry-picking is the purposeful selection of certain data that support a hypothesis or key research question, while ignoring the data that do not. Maybe researchers start crossing out the information gathered in a survey because it just doesn't fit the results they wanted—justifying that practice because in retrospect those individuals were thought to be too old, or too young, or the wrong shape or gender for the experiment. Or maybe they don't justify it at all, assuming no one will ever know. Until someone else attempts to repeat the study, it's difficult for a layperson or even another scientist to spot tainted results.

One diet guru who based his work on science—but came to be known as a cherry picker in some circles—was Ancel Keys. Keys was known for developing "K-rations" (military food packages first used in World War II) and later, popularizing the Mediterranean diet, which focuses on lean meats, fruits and vegetables, and olive oil. In 1959, Keys and his wife Margaret published *Eat Well and Stay Well,* a cookbook that promoted the Mediterranean diet and implicated saturated fat in cardiovascular disease. He based his recommendations on a review of existing information from many studies in several countries around the world, correlating saturated fat intake with the incidence of cardiovascular disease. This became his infamous "Seven Countries Study," which produced an anti-fat hypothesis—an idea that the food industry embraced.

In the Seven Countries Study, Keys produced graphs that were clear, stark, and disturbing, showing a rapid increase in the incidence of heart disease with increased saturated fat intake. Implicated were everything from big beef burgers to pork chops, bacon, and sour cream. Foods containing saturated fats and dietary cholesterol were under attack. Results were widely accepted by the scientific community, the food industry, and interested people—including myself. The data seemed compelling, and the conclusion even more so: eat less fat and more plant matter for weight management and health. The American Heart Association, which had formed early in the twentieth century, gained momentum with Keys's claims, and heavily promoted the low-fat directive with media messages and recipes representing "heart-friendly food." The food industry proceeded to create a plethora of low-fat food products that, incidentally, were also high-sugar—but Keys's data showed no problem with sugar consumption.

Since then, vocal critics have argued that Keys was highly selective with his data, especially by ignoring countries that did not fit the high saturated fat/high cardiovascular disease pattern. This argument about the misrepresentation of science is presented in numerous scholarly critiques, including pediatric endocrinologist Robert Lustig's virally popular lecture, "Sugar: The Bitter Truth," and his book, *Fat Chance: Beating the Odds against Sugar, Processed Food, Obesity, and Disease.*

The well-known Framingham Study eventually accumulated data that addressed Keys's views, with the director, physician William Castelli, reporting in 1992: "In Framingham, Mass, the more saturated fat one ate, the more cholesterol one ate, the *more calories one ate,* the lower the person's serum cholesterol." Numerous Framingham research reports and other studies since then continue to offer new insights. Nevertheless, there is general agreement that there were risk factors in play other than dietary cholesterol intake—total calories and sugar intake, for example.

Clearly, figuring out the science behind food is incredibly complex. So how do we as FoodWISE eaters separate the truth from the hype? Scientific study itself has much to tell us, but when pundits take the information and run with it, parsing out the truth becomes a much bigger challenge. Our best tool: an assertive, questioning attitude. Becoming FoodWISE means absorbing as much wisdom as we can, from as many different sources as possible. But we have to accept that it's impossible to keep track of every study about some aspect of food, nutrition, or diet that we're interested in.

For me it's a question of finding a balance between a level of informed understanding that I feel comfortable with, and the practical need to avoid getting completely bogged down in every difficult question I encounter. Still, I enjoy following contemporary scientists and their work (which I provide examples of and fully discuss later)—whether it is theoretical, based in clinical studies, or derived from experiments. I may not agree with the results, but I appreciate the different approaches. Each provides something the others do not, giving me multiple ways to look at the world. Finally, I have to think about what works for my FoodWISE life. The balance is different for everyone, but finding it is essential to becoming a FoodWISE eater.

It's clear that understanding what the best science can tell us is essential to making sensible food choices. And figuring out what that information is for ourselves is essential to our FoodWISE approach to making choices: taking control of our own decision-making about food.

To illustrate how we can review complicated scientific information and come to our own conclusions, let's look at particular work on three topics that get attention in the food world and are important in our food choices: saturated fats (in the "Fats to the Rescue?" section), sugar (in the "Carbohydrates and the Problem of Fructose" section), and taste combined with food quality considerations (in the "Sensory Science" section). This work is particularly interesting because some of the findings are counterintuitive, go against the common wisdom, and are unexpected. There's nothing like provocative results to stir you to dig deeper.

Protein, Fats, Carbs: The Components of Food

First, let's dig a little deeper into the science of food itself, before we spread out again to see what science tells us about how we should eat and what our bodies need.

As far as the body is concerned, food has three major components: proteins, fats, and carbohydrates (and under the carb umbrella, all sugars). That's it: everything we eat belongs to one of these groups, or (most often) is made up of two or three in varying proportions. Each group has a different chemical composition, is processed differently by the body, and does different work.

Of the three components, protein might be the least controversial. Before we dive into the complicated belief structures surrounding fats and carbohydrates, it's worth discussing protein a little: What exactly is it? What does it do?

Proteins are critically important for virtually all aspects of our human functioning—the structure of our skeletons, the elasticity of our skin (the body's largest organ), blood, enzymes, antibodies, hormones. We need a wide array of amino acids—the building blocks of proteins—in order to function. Neurotransmitters, like serotonin and dopamine, are all built of amino acids combined into proteins.

Despite what manufacturers of high-protein shakes, bars, and supplements might want us to believe, it's actually not difficult for the average person to get enough protein, so long as she or he is consuming enough calories in general. (Calories are a measure of the energy produced by any kind of food.) Because of this, and because few people have demonized protein (yet!), we don't need to spend too much time on it here. Suffice it to say that, while some false beliefs about protein are out there (think health "halos" around sweet protein sugar drinks), most people probably aren't surprised to hear that sufficient protein is a good thing. It's those other two elements of our diets that we seem to have so much trouble understanding: fats and carbs.

Fats to the Rescue? Debunking Stories about Cholesterol

High-fat diets increase cholesterol, right? And high cholesterol leads to heart disease, right? Which means cholesterol, and by extension fats, should be avoided at all costs, right? This is the popular understanding of cholesterol, and a big part of the reason why so many low-fat/sugary/highly processed foods, "low in cholesterol," fill our grocery store shelves and our pantries.

Yes, cholesterol levels are related to what we eat, among other factors. The stories—journalistic and scientific alike—about cholesterol are conflicting, and sometimes misleading. Before we can begin to understand and question what we hear, it helps to get some basic information straight. What *are* dietary "fats," exactly? And what is cholesterol? Many modern diet devotees may be surprised to learn that we *wouldn't* be better off without either one.

First, what is fat? Fats are composed of fatty acids, and there are usually three subunits for each fat ("fat" and "fatty acids" are often used interchangeably, even though "fatty acids" are a subset of "fat"). Three fatty acid subunits bound together are a triglyceride. They are joined by another molecule, called glycerol, at the top.

Saturated fats have no double bonds in their component fatty acids—they are "saturated" with hydrogen (which has implications for their ability to react chemically). The important thing for our purposes here is that they tend to be solid at room temperature. They are found in animal foods, eggs, dairy, meat, and palm and coconut oils.

Unsaturated fats—fats that do have those double bonds—are generally found in foods from plants. These contain the fats that liquefy easily and tend to be liquid at room temperature. Monounsaturated fats have *one* double bond in their component fatty acids. Polyunsaturated fats have more than one double bond in their component fatty acids. Although liquid at room temperature, they can start to solidify at cooler temperatures. Versatile olive oil, which we will be talking about later in this section, contains mostly mono-unsaturated fatty acids. Oils high in polyunsaturated fats include many vegetable oils such as soy, corn, and sunflower. Fish such as salmon, mackerel, herring, and trout also contain polyunsaturated fats.

Two polyunsaturated fatty acids are of particular interest: omega-3 and omega-6. These cannot be manufactured by the body, but they are needed and so must be consumed daily. They are "essential" in that they are critical components of cell membranes, and play a role in the body's anti-inflammatory responses and blood cholesterol chemistry. Michael Pollan wrote of these critical fatty acids in *The Omnivore's Dilemma*. In our Western diets, he writes, we get a good amount of omega-6 fatty acids, but omega-3s, equally essential, are gravely lacking. These fatty acids are found mostly in the oils of particular marine fish (salmon, sardines), although walnuts and flaxseeds contain a dose as well. The actual kind of omega-3 varies depending on the source.

Most Americans are far more likely to consume foods that contain omega-6, such as nuts, corn, and other seeds, and the oils made from each. Omega-6 is important, but Pollan is concerned that we are over-consuming corn (and soy) in all the snack foods that we eat, meaning we're not getting a good balance of different fatty acids. Reportedly, pre–industrial era diets had ratios of omega-6 to omega-3 fats of about 1:1, quite a contrast to the top-heavy 16:1 to 20:1 of our contemporary grain-fed beef-based diets. We'll talk more about the benefits of fats in a moment.

Another type of fat, trans fats, is hard to find in natural environments. Trans fats are in the guts of some animals, but that's about it. It was the discovery and use of a hydrogenation process in the twentieth century, coupled with relatively cheap substrates—corn and soy, that led to the creation of artificial trans fats in margarine and other products substituting for butter, lard, and tallow. Trans fats can change both the taste and texture of foods, and are used to make them more acceptable. But what is more acceptable to the consumer—more rich tasting? more fatty tasting? It's hard to find literature that explains clearly what that taste is, but the industry certainly believes people like it.

The trans fats that we are likely to encounter in our food supply, then, come from industrial-made processed foods manufactured with partially hydrogenated oils. I refer to these trans fats as "processed fats." These, of all the types of fat, are the ones our bodies are least equipped to deal with— which makes sense, since trans fats are mostly a recent human invention. Food companies have caught on to this in their advertising: just keep a count of "zero trans fat" labels next time you're at the grocery store. The trouble is, "zero" seems to be used loosely here; cookies, chips, and cake mixes that purport to be trans fat–free can still contain far more of the substance than we need. Cutting all fat out of the diet doesn't make sense, as we'll see in just a moment. Processed fat, though, does seem to be something we have too much of.

Fats are complex; they and their relationship to our bodies are not as straightforward as those of us who believe that "fats make us fat" would think. But what about cholesterol? Surely we haven't been oversimplifying that, too?

Well, probably so. Many people do already know that there are two main types of cholesterol. HDL cholesterol, which means high-density lipoprotein, doesn't actually contribute to heart disease at all. If cholesterol and heart disease are linked, it's LDL (low-density lipoprotein) cholesterol that's the culprit—particularly the small-molecule variety. If we eliminate saturated fats, as many diets tell us we must do in order to cut down on "bad" cholesterol, we're actually cutting other types of cholesterol from our diet— and our bodies won't be happy. It's the consumption of saturated fats that enables our bodies to convert that small-molecule LDL cholesterol into the large-molecule kind. Once those molecules get bigger, even LDL cholesterol doesn't seem to be a big factor in heart disease. As for HDL, most of us need more of it. Further, cholesterol is an important building block for hormones and neurotransmitters, and it's essential for vitamin absorption. Cholesterol is a precursor to vitamin D. Without it in our diet, our vitamin D levels would probably take a dive.

An example of innovative thinking is the path of computer engineer Stephanie Seneff's theoretical investigations into how all this works. Seneff's interest in food was catalyzed by a medical situation, when her spouse was prescribed statins, a cholesterol-lowering medication. This led her to look into the effect of statins on cholesterol, whether we needed that waxy, fat-like substance at all, and what the connections were between saturated fat and cholesterol. Seneff has reported on her findings and proposed that many debilitating diseases result from a lack of saturated fats in the diet, as well as deficiencies in vitamin D, sulfur, and cholesterol; and that a lack of sun exposure (key in the production of both cholesterol sulfate and vitamin D) makes things worse.

Early on, Seneff read that statins could indeed reduce a high blood serum cholesterol. And yet, the reported side effects were troublesome. Severe muscle damage caused by statins could lead to muscle pain and weakness, as well as a life-threatening condition called rhabdomyolysis. Worse, the depletion of cholesterol supply from the liver to the tissues leads to cell membrane dysfunction, systemically; and possibly to severe problems like diabetes, heart failure, cancer, dementia, and even Lou Gehrig's disease. Statin drugs essentially make a person age at an accelerated rate, primarily due to the absence of cholesterol and other vital compounds whose production statins impair.

Seneff came away from her studies with a conclusion that many probably found surprising. Her path to good health: bring on the bacon. Fats make our bodies function better. For those of us worried about weight gain, sugar is the culprit, not saturated fat and cholesterol. Seneff argues that lifestyle changes over the past forty years, in particular cutting back on sun exposure and dietary fat, have done us harm. But many of us have come to believe that avoiding these things is "healthy."

Part of the problem, too, Seneff says, is our large intake of refined carbohydrates (i.e., highly processed and sugary foods that digest quickly and cause blood sugar to spike). Repeatedly and over time, this leads to insulin resistance and, quite possibly, Type 2 diabetes, part of what's often referred to as "the metabolic syndrome" associated with high weight and abdominal fat. That belly fat is a form of fat that simply does not perform the same protective functions as subcutaneous fat throughout the body. Belly fat is, in effect, the unnecessary fat we gain not from eating fat *per se,* but from eating too many carbohydrates. Further, that belly fat is in the wrong place to do us any good by protecting organs. How ironic, that belly fat is actually a signal that we have insufficient saturated fat in our diets!

So, wait—eating fat is good? Doesn't this go against everything we're told? Maybe this is a moment to stop—think—then act. Take a look at Seneff's process: she is trained in using scientific principles and has applied them to her study of nutrition and disease. Importantly, she is selling nothing. She simply studies metabolic pathways to see what effect each food really has, checking to see if there is a strong theoretical base for understanding a particular biochemistry pathway or mechanism. Once fat enters the body, what does it actually do?

To put it briefly, Seneff believes that obesity is the consequence of eating too little saturated fat (and too many sugary carbs), and that the fat accumulation we see with obesity is actually the body trying to compensate for not enough saturated fat in the diet. Obesity and the metabolic syndrome shown in abdominal weight gain and high levels of LDL cholesterol and circulating blood triglycerides, high blood sugar, and high blood pressure, may be the body's way of building massive fat cells in an attempt to provide needed fat for essential body processes. Further, what we call "heart disease" may actually be the body creating cholesterol deposits, as a silo or reservoir, close to the heart muscle, because no natural, safe form of cholesterol is available, and the heart critically depends on sufficient cholesterol to function properly. Whew, this *is* a shift in thinking!

We need a certain amount of fat—not belly fat, but body fat that protects and fuels essential organs. Stay too thin, and you might sacrifice brain development as well as the integrity of the myelin sheath coating the nerve fibers. Those sheaths are entirely made up of lipids, as are the membranes of other cells—and the body will hoard cholesterol to ensure their proper functioning. The body will draw from every system, to remove life-giving cholesterol and fatty acids—from joints, for example, and arthritis results; from the central nervous system, and multiple sclerosis results; from the brain, and Alzheimer's results—this is what Seneff is theorizing. Perhaps our bodies are outsmarting us in our decisions to go on low-fat diets.

Researchers argue that fat is so dynamic it can be considered an endocrine organ itself, releasing hormones and proteins that, with the adrenal and thyroid glands, orchestrate many important bodily functions. The idea here is that fat, rather than being an inert tissue, actually is highly active and exerts an influence on the whole-body metabolism. Perhaps this makes something like cheese (high in cholesterol and saturated fat) a perfect food.

It all sounds complicated—it is complicated! But the discussion keeps coming back to those saturated fats and whole foods that haven't been chemically treated. Seneff is not clear as to how much cholesterol and saturated fat we need. There is no formula. Their functionality is also related to various additional dietary elements. Seneff believes that the best source of these (or any) nutrients is organic whole foods, minimally processed. For many of us, this means a lifestyle change, and that can sometimes be difficult to face.

Seneff isn't an experimental researcher or diet guru. Yet she, in full Food-WISE spirit, tells stories that she believes need to be told—even if they aren't what we expect to hear. My retelling of those stories is part of information-rich FoodWISE thinking. It is up to us to figure out how we ourselves can act on what she's suggested—if only to reconsider those processed "low-fat" carbs so many commercial diet programs have convinced us we need.

Carbohydrates and the Problem of Fructose

What *about* those carbs? Just as we did with fats, let's start by seeing what exactly a carbohydrate is. Carbohydrates can be found as sugars but also in more complex forms. Sugars like glucose and fructose are known as "monosaccharides" or single sugars; sugars like sucrose (regular table sugar) or lactose (found in milk) are known as "disaccharides" or double sugars. Each sucrose molecule is composed of two single sugars—one glucose and one fructose. The third major category of carbohydrate (single and double sugars being the first two) is complex carbohydrates. These consist of more complex forms like starches and fiber typically found in vegetables like potatoes and corn (but also in whole and refined grains).

Just as with fats, cutting out carbs altogether isn't a safe solution to whatever we think our dietary problems are. But we should be mindful of what kinds of carbs we consume. Enter Robert Lustig, whose work in pediatric neuroendocrinology centers around an ingredient you can probably find in almost every processed juice or condiment in your fridge—fructose. Sucrose or table sugar is in many of our foods, and, as I just mentioned, half of each sucrose molecule is fructose. We eat a lot of sugar, and that means we eat a lot of fructose. We also eat a lot of high fructose corn syrup (HFCS), a cheap sweetener that's about 20% sweeter than white table sugar. According to Lustig, that sweetener may be the source of a lot of our health problems.

Estimates of past and present sugar consumption vary. Two hundred years ago Americans, on average, ate perhaps two to four pounds of added sugar a year. Now we eat, by one estimate, 17 teaspoons (about 71 grams) daily or about 57 pounds each year, or by another estimate about 152 pounds per year. Don't worry about which estimate is more accurate—both are alarming. Recommendations from groups such as the World Health Organization are to reduce intake, for adults, to no more than one-third to one-half our current consumption.

Lustig's research addresses many questions, one of which is: What happens to us when we consume fructose, that sweet molecule in table sugar? Fructose is metabolized like no other sugar, breaking down almost completely in the liver. What is not immediately burned can be instead turned into liver fat, with lasting effects. This is one reason why Lustig makes the analogy, "You would never give your child a can of beer but you don't think twice about giving [her/him] a can of soda." According to Lustig, fructose and alcohol are metabolized almost identically in the liver. This means that chronic fructose exposure can cause diseases similar to chronic ethanol exposure: fatty liver disease, hypertension, fetal insulin resistance, and, if not addiction, then at least habituation. We get used to it, and we want more and more.

In his lecture video "Sugar: The Bitter Truth" and book, *Fat Chance*, Lustig explains how the body metabolizes fructose. All fructose, whether it be high fructose corn syrup in bread or fructose in maple syrup, is powerfully sweet—and, as it turns out, virtually addictive. I don't use that term lightly; the body of scientific evidence certainly points in this direction. The idea of a "sugar high" is spot on, especially when fructose is the sugar in question. Fructose molecules go straight to the liver, and instead of being put to good use as immediate energy, those molecules mostly end up as fat. Remember Seneff's claims about carbs and weight gain? Lustig wholeheartedly agrees. Fructose builds up as useless fat in the body, engorging the liver without helping any of the body's other organs the way consuming actual fats might. Fructose in excess also interferes with normal hormonal communication within the body to stop eating. And if that's not enough, fructose drives insulin resistance, leading to a condition called hyperinsulinemia, or "too much insulin" in comparison with the amount of available glucose. Lustig unabashedly makes a causal connection between over-consumption of fructose and metabolic disease.

Lustig's bottom line: limit sugar consumption. In the real world that means avoiding most processed foods, since high fructose corn syrup or sucrose turn up in everything from jelly to supermarket bread. The marginally good news: some whole food sugars do exist. Molasses—mostly a by-product of sugarcane refining—for instance, is high in glucose. But it's not very sweet, and so is less acceptable to many.

In the 1970s, cheap sugar sweeteners, and eventually HFCS, found their way into everything. And it wasn't just a one-to-one substitution of corn sweeteners (fructose) for white cane and beet sugar (sucrose). Not only did the type of sugar we were eating change, we also started eating more of it. It was part of what happened with eating fewer whole foods. The heavy fructose load in processed foods also meant less fibrous carbohydrates (which, incidentally, did not freeze well in processed foods anyway). Further, in the process, partially hydrogenated or trans fats are substituted for saturated fat.

So, thanks to fructose, we're losing nutrients we need—fiber and saturated fats—and instead consuming food that leads to weight gain and insulin spikes. When spikes occur, the brain doesn't get the leptin signal—high insulin levels reduce leptin signaling in the brain, which is interpreted as "brain starvation." That means we keep eating and making new fat—and not breaking down the old fat. And since fructose doesn't suppress the hunger hormone ghrelin either, we still "feel" hungry after eating a Twinkie or ten. That's right. You don't feel as full after eating fructose (even compared to the exact same amount of calories as glucose), since ghrelin levels stay high.

Fiber is part of the equation. Where there is fructose in nature, there are also copious amounts of fiber (think sugarcane, with a stalk that's all fiber). Eating fiber with fructose helps us to feel like we've actually eaten. This means we are most likely to overeat when we eat fructose that's had the fiber processed right out of it—like fruit juice.

As Lustig acknowledges in his 2017 book, *The Hacking of the American Mind: The Science Behind the Corporate Takeover of Our Bodies and Brains,* avoiding fructose is not easy. The anti-fructose believers among us have to fight industry's driving message: buy this and you'll be happy. And it's that promise—happiness—that ropes in so many of us.

The Joys of Sugar: Dopamine, Serotonin, and Our Addiction to Fructose

Lustig firmly believes that ours is a culture of addiction and depression—and fructose is the "cheapest thrill." We give a thrill-making substance—juice— to babies without a second thought. Patterns are established and chronic disease can ultimately result. One important piece to this is that the major "reward" neurotransmitter in our brains, dopamine, is readily available in our fructose culture. And fructose, like every substance or behavior that releases substantial amounts of dopamine, can quickly lead to dopamine addiction. Well … is that so bad? What's wrong with so much pleasure? The problem is, dopamine has a dark side. The more dopamine we have, the less serotonin our brains produce, and serotonin is the "contentment" neu-rotransmitter. This transmitter is supposed to tell our brains that in fact we don't need any more of what we think we need. Importantly, deficiencies in serotonin lead quickly to depression.

Lustig explains that the one thing that gets in the way of serotonin-related contentment is dopamine. This means that not only does dopamine pleasure fail to give you any long-term happiness, but it actually prevents it. So the more pleasure you seek, the more unhappy (or, literally, less happy) you get. It's easy to see how modern society, loaded with the easy quick fixes of sugary processed foods, is hooked on this entire process of *unhappiness*— unhappiness in the pursuit of pleasure.

By contrast, we eat for happiness when we nourish our bodies with good food, while simultaneously making food choices that economically and envi-ronmentally support the communities in which we live. This allows us to be the best we can be, and therefore to be happy. The problem is that when we focus too much on the pleasure of eating, we will be tempted to seek it in the simple chemical satisfaction of things like sugar. While this may provide us with a rush of pleasure right then, it undermines the nourishment that will make us happy in the long run.

Lustig and I are kindred spirits; we agree that the cooking he talks about as an antidote to quick-pleasure-seeking is a fundamental part of gastronomical contentment. Cooking your own food ensures that you know what you are eating, that it is whole food, and also that it is Wise in other ways. This means that it can be delicious, sustainable, and ethical. This kind of eating experience is what will promote lasting happiness. High fructose and unhealthy processed-fat–laden fast food give us nothing but, literally, unhappiness (and, literally, cheap thrills).

The food industry has always known what it was doing (in terms of selling processed fat and sugar) with its extensive product research and development efforts. Researchers found a clear paper trail showing that the sugar industry in the 1960s paid some Harvard scientists to essentially publish a review of cherry-picked studies that minimized the role of sugar in heart disease and shifted the blame to fat. Other examples of industry-slanted research keep coming to light from time to time.

Lustig wonders if we couldn't lower our national price tag for health care by focusing more on food reform. Food reform means fewer convenience carbohydrates—that is, less processed food. Yet as long as a market exists for these process-intensive, fructose-heavy foods, eliminating fructose is going to be a difficult task. Indeed, becoming FoodWISE could mean taking a personal role in this shift, as more and more people transition their lifestyles away from fructose and toward whole foods.

This transition conforms to Lustig's conclusions, and Stephanie Seneff's as well. When it comes to the practical question of "What should you eat?" the answer is pretty clear. Whole foods: no processed sugar added in, no saturated fats taken out (or substituted for). This fundamental component of FoodWISE eating seems to be the surest path toward physical nourishment, prolonged well-being, and, ultimately, happiness.

Sensory Science: The Taste Experience

With all the research we've been discussing that suggests a FoodWISE lifestyle is worth considering, it seems like it would be easy to just cut processed foods out of our lives. If we've learned anything from Lustig, though, it's that we eat processed foods for a reason: our brains latch onto that sugar, even though it ultimately does us harm. For many of us, transitioning to whole foods will mean retraining ourselves, down to our very taste buds. What is "good" food, really? Moving beyond the quick "bliss point" provided by processed fat-sugar-salt combinations, how can we teach ourselves to find more lasting pleasure in whole foods?

Much of it comes down to taste. There's actually an entire branch of science devoted to taste. It's called sensory analysis (or sensory evaluation) and it studies a lot more than taste: sight, smell, touch, and more. Among other things, the field examines how we—consumers—perceive food. It recognizes that it's not just tea tasters and cheesemakers and sommeliers who have a good (or definitive) sensory perception of food and drink; it's also the rest of us, just regular consumers. I'm sure you can foresee where industry could—and does—go with this: Much of the research in sensory science is industry-funded. Certainly, the research tends to be oriented toward practical applications. Early on, for example, it sought to help provide sufficient nutrition to troops serving overseas in World War II. Part of the question was, what food tastes good? This is about the time that sensory science began to evolve from the larger discipline of food science.

Usually, industrialized agriculture and food manufacturing companies have been the beneficiaries of sensory science. They want to sell a product, and want to know what it is about the product that consumers like and what will make them want to buy it. In this role, sensory science could be seen as only about selling a product, addressing a specific industry's or company's competitive edge.

But to my FoodWISE thinking, the information from this science can help us understand a lot about food quality—what is a good food, or, what do we perceive as a good food, and why. These questions are important.

Like advertising and all the other messages we receive, our sensory perceptions help determine what foods we like and therefore what our food choices will be. The findings of sensory science can help us understand our perceptions about food.

Remember those flavorful tomatoes I harvested on the Amish farm? What do you think made those tomatoes so good? Heritage varieties, sunshine, good soil, and farmer–plant connections, of course. For University of Florence sensory food scientists Erminio Monteleone and Caterina Dinnella, however, there's a lot going on with how those formative elements are expressed in the tomatoes themselves.

Our ability to sense the sweet, sour, bitter, salty, and umami (think soy sauce—it's the taste of the amino acid glutamine) components of food comprises taste. Flavor combines our sense of these inputs with our olfactory or smell system. For right now, we'll stick with taste sensations.

Of course, we don't think about any of this when we bite into a ripe tomato. Those heritage tomatoes contain a nice mix of sugars, acids, and volatile compounds—maybe fifteen to twenty actors in all. Beta ionone provides a lot of flavor, as well as that classic tomato smell. There's also a high concentration of vitamin C. It's one thing to know the chemical components; it is quite another to be able to taste them (or even some of them), and to identify a food by that taste.

What I find interesting is where this science can lead. Researchers study consumers' perceptions of foods from artisanal production systems—which, going back to our discussions of FoodWISE agriculture in Part 1, come from a variety of types of farms. Researchers also study the factors influencing consumer preferences for fresh rather than processed foods.

The study of artisanal foods (foods from very localized areas and small-batch production, inevitably made a bit differently each time) presents challenges for sensory scientists, particularly in controlled settings. Highly standardized, industrial-style foods are ready-made, so to speak, for such studies. Trying to sort out what makes a consumer reliably like a food is not difficult in a laboratory setting, where you can control for other variables, and use standardized foods. Artisanal foods, on the other hand, can vary dramatically from day to day and season to season.

Sensory scientist Jacob Lahne considers the validity of the methods ("best practices") for conducting such research. Lahne, like other sensory scientists, is interested in what constitutes a "true" sensory experience. He calls for more careful attention to what we mean by valid sensory properties attributed to specific practices and locales (what about that slight green tinge to Butte County, Sacramento Valley early-season olive oil)? And whether or not we can get valid descriptions of food when we take it out of a production context and put it in a laboratory setting. These are good questions to ask of the overcommercialized, standardized market we are in today. In order to move away from processed foods, we need to understand what we're moving toward—and why our tomato sauce will be so much better once we get there. For that, we need to study the olive oil as well as the tomatoes that make good sauce.

Monteleone and Dinnella have shared some of their knowledge with my students in summer classes in Italy. Their research includes sensory responses, as well as hedonic (whether it's pleasurable or not) consumer responses, to foods. This is important information when you're trying to find out, for example, what the reasons are for people not eating more fresh vegetables. Another aspect of their work is looking at how information about the origins (and also the health properties) of food affects consumer responses.

The work of Monteleone and Dinnella shows that exposure to different kinds of food matters. They argue that our innate ability to use taste to determine what foods we do and do not need exists only at a very basic level, applying to basic macronutrient components but not to more sophisticated flavors or overall food quality. They suggest that we will never be able to recognize a high-quality oil—or cheese, or wine—unless we expose our taste buds to it consistently and often. If we don't eat a diversity of foods, we might lose the ability to distinguish unique tastes and differing qualities.

Not only does this mean we will miss out on specific nutrient benefits that, for example, virgin olive oil has and cheap, processed, rancid oil doesn't. It also means that, gradually, variety will leak out of our diets, leaving us with a lot of processed foods that all taste pretty much the same. Bland? Boring? That is when we reach for the sugar or the salt, relying more and more on processed condiments to add some punch to what we're eating. Subtle flavors are getting processed out of our foods and, without exposure to these flavors, most of us don't even know what we're missing.

The case of olive oil can illustrate taste scientists' points. Olive oil is a perfectly whole food. It has been pressed, of course, but the *whole fruit* has been pressed, a very different process from the one used to extract other oils. Sunflower and safflower oils, for example, come from seeds and often are extracted with solvents, deodorized, and generally processed much more intensively. This means that when we buy "pure" virgin olive oil, actual olive oil is what we're getting.

When thinking about quality, taste scientists look at the intersection between what is "claimed about the product and what is actually offered to the consumer." An excellent extra virgin olive oil must meet defined standards (which may not translate directly into what the consumer tastes): levels of acidity, and presence of certain chemicals like free fatty acids. So must other grades of oil: virgin olive oil, olive pomace oil (extracted from the pulpy residue, usually with solvents), and so on. Many factors affect the quality ranking of an olive oil, such as the traceability of the producer and processor, the ripeness of the olive, and how closely the pressing follows harvesting. How long is the oil in contact with the crushed olive paste and in what temperature conditions? Is the oil made from a single cultivar of olives, or a variety? Further, each country may have different standards to achieve a particular grade.

In addition to quantifiable characteristics that measurably affect an oil's physical quality, oils are judged based on their "sensory profile"—different component tastes that make up their overall flavor. This is evaluated in terms of "sensory performance" or functionality, basically a question of, for example, how the flavor shows up in cooking. Perhaps an olive oil that is pungent and burns the back of the throat on its own can in fact brighten and sweeten an entire tomato sauce—we've talked about this already. We consumers are no longer used to this kind of oil, though; we expect the more readily available, cheaper, bland, and even rancid versions. Perhaps the more we learn about food, by becoming more informed and experienced, the more we can understand the true nutritious and culinary potential of what's in our kitchens.

The application of taste science exists in an interesting space, a sort of bridging link. On the one hand, there's the FoodWISE goal of producing and valuing a diversity of sensations that can be present in a food. On the other is the driving interest of business to standardize around simple, satisfying, and familiar flavors. Have you ever seen the green beans displayed at a county fair, where the first place entries are completely uniform in length, shape, and color? Likewise, in international competitions, oils are valued for their ability to be what industry calls "balanced" (so, no harsh tastes) on their own, rather than with consideration of what's appropriate for specific dishes. This trend toward uniformity means we lose the culture surrounding particular foods—and industry promotes this loss.

It seems clear that if the sensory performance of something like olive oil is so important, we need to know more about it. Maybe that means forming partnerships among producers and distributors and retail food businesses. And that should include the chefs (and cooks) who use olive oil in specific dishes. Of course, this idea does not apply just to olive oil. Cheeses come to mind, but so do fresh fruits and vegetables in various stages of maturity. A completely new world of flavor possibilities remains to be discovered by those who explore, experiment, and become FoodWISE eaters. But then again, this is Monteleone and Dinnella's point: taste and flavor are important. Our senses help form our concepts of food quality, determine our enjoyment of foods, and ultimately influence our food choices. Trying a variety of foods, and similar foods at different stages of ripeness and processing, is how we educate our senses.

Closing Thoughts: Practicing FoodWISE for Life

My students sometimes wonder where I stand on food. They wonder if I am a low-fat devotee or a vegetarian or a raw-foods missionary. Really, I am a proponent of one thing: mindful eating of mostly whole foods.

I like to know where my food comes from, I like to think about the field or farm or farmer or fisher when I'm eating the food; I feel better knowing about those places and people. I believe that a main goal in life is to not be too hungry, but also to not overeat. In a house of teens, there was always that temptation, with so much food around. I am selective about my sweets, but am especially fond of raw chocolate's velvety texture. I believe unprocessed food is a good food choice. I believe in slow food—food that is *good*-tasting, *clean* and efficient (in terms of few wastes produced), and *fair* to all two- and four-legged beings, as well as those with fins. I didn't coin the *good-clean-fair* mantra; *Slow Food Nation* author Carlo Petrini did. I build on his ideas.

In the Introduction, I talked about what I consider high-quality foods. For me, these include crisp beans, fresh eggs, and wild-caught meat—all part of the FoodWISE experience. Why? Because all of these foods are loaded with tastes that I miss by just going to a supermarket.

But I also pick up pasta sauce, someone else's fresh pasta, canned beans, and canned tomatoes—even rice in a prepared boiling bag—off the supermarket shelves. I'm fond of take-away raw sourdough from my local wood-fired pizza restaurant (then I make the pizza at home). I also enjoy sit-down eating at that same restaurant with a group. Here, too, I taste quality: the pasta sauce that's low in sugar, the greens that are fresh.

Inevitably I write all this from the perspective of my own set of beliefs about food. There's no way I can escape the formative impact of those elaborate dinners my mother made for our extended Italian family and friends, or the hours she spent daily in the kitchen preparing tasty and varied meals for us.

What you yourself think is the ideal breakfast will have been shaped by whether you had bacon, ham, or scrapple with an egg every morning, or absorbed the message from years of warnings about the perils of eggs and whole milk. How much home cooking you saw may affect your own interest in doing it—for better or worse.

I hope this part of the book has helped you acknowledge and work through some of what affects your food choices. We've explored the influence of food beliefs and advertising and the roles diets and popular culture play in dictating what we eat and how. Using the lens of science, we've looked at how limiting calories, especially when they are in whole foods, is not an answer to anything; and what might happen in our bodies when we choose primarily low-fat high-sugar foods. At this point, you understand a lot more about what goes on with your food—from the farms that grow it, to the companies that sell it, to what you stir into your own pot.

Everyone's FoodWISE journey will be different, but I hope you can incorporate what I've given you here. Bring back the fats. Cut back on carbs, especially the processed ones. Everything our bodies need is already present in the whole foods around us. It's only when we start messing with those foods—taking out the fat, adding in the preservatives; taking the "whole" out of the grains and putting in artificial vitamins instead; bringing on the sugar and salt to make up for everything we're taking away—that our bodies run into trouble. That's when we start to put on the belly fat, as some believe, due to deficits of saturated fat. For me, it's worth the effort to sit down with research results that may not be what we want to hear, but do offer interesting ideas for a wholesome future.

So, I ask: Why not try out new things, change our food choices, and watch the effects on our well-being and appetite and how we feel in our bodies? If your answer is, "Yes, why not?" it's probably time to continue on to Part 3, where the principles of FoodWISE will show us how to actually put these ideas into practice in ways that are Whole, Informed, Sustainable, and develop Experience-based thinking. Let's figure out how to live with empathy for our planet, and for the organisms most directly in our care: ourselves.

PART 3

FoodWISE: Choosing Experience

W e've considered a lot of different factors at play in our food choices. Now it's time to put it all into action. Experiencing FoodWISE seals the deal. In the Introduction, I described FoodWISE guidelines as questions around how Whole, Informed, Sustainable, and Experience can guide our food choices. We looked at threats to a Whole and Sustainable agricultural web in Part 1, and challenges in making Informed food choices in Part 2, so let's now bring Experience to FoodWISE thinking.

First, let's take a quick look at where we've been. The Introduction was FoodWISE Ground Zero. Everybody eats; but is our food whole? How is it processed? Who's selling it to us, anyway? And are our beliefs about it fierce, unwavering? In Part 1, we looked at FoodWISE in our shared world—and that raised issues of access, resources, incentives, resilience, and community. In Part 2 we got personal, looking at food in the way we know it best, thinking about our own food beliefs, emotions, and how advertising affects the way we eat. Part 2 also took us into science, suggesting what information we might pay attention to, and why. Now it's time to bring it all together: Living FoodWISE is making Whole-food and Whole-farm choices. Given what we now know as informed consumers, where do we go from here? Ultimately, we'll go to recipes in Part 4 for examples of delicious whole foods, and if the ingredients are the result of Whole-farm systems, all the better.

FOODWISE REVIEW

In the Introduction, I talked about our complex food system being an agricultural web. All the activities of growing, processing, selling, and consuming food are interwoven threads of the web. All the farms, grain mills, packing plants, grocery stores, and home kitchens are points where these threads intersect. All the farmers, millers, butchers, bakers, grocery clerks, and cooks are the people who inhabit the web—making it work, and depending on it for their sustenance and livelihood.

If one thread weakens or breaks, disruptions spread and potentially affect the entire web. A drought or disease outbreak that reduces farm production, a transportation breakdown or cut-off in labor supply, a change in nutrition assistance programs—all these disruptions affect businesses, activities, and ultimately people everywhere in the all-encompassing agricultural web. We are all part of this web—because we all eat. In our personal worlds, if we don't have access to whole food, we are vulnerable.

So, in Part 3, we begin with a review of our FoodWISE guidelines. How can Whole, Informed, Sustainable, and Experience-based thinking guide our food choices toward Whole foods and Whole farms?

Whole Foods

As we discussed in the Introduction, whole foods generally means minimal processing. If little is taken away and nothing is added, the food is still functionally whole in terms of nutrients. This means choosing whole grains rather than refined flours; fish and pasture-fed livestock; and dishes that are rich in fruits, vegetables, and beans. The key to maintaining food wholeness is that no unwanted chemicals are introduced to enhance flavor, appearance, or shelf life. And in Part 1, we asked the question, is the farm that produced it Whole, too? Is it part of an integrated agricultural system producing crops and livestock, recycling wastes, and connecting to consumers?

Fats

In looking at nutrients, we started with fats (after acknowledging that proteins aren't very controversial, as long as we're not overconsuming them).

Whole foods have the fats our bodies need—for example, in helping to increase fat-soluble vitamin absorption. They literally support our organs and bones, providing cushioning and helping us absorb vitamins. From Stephanie Seneff's theoretical work in Part 2, we learned that fats may be important in preventing deficiencies in cholesterol. This doesn't mean we should overeat fats, even when they're in a whole food coming from an integrated farm or free-range chicken yard or ecologically intact marine system. But it's a good idea, based on the information we've reviewed, to include some fats in our meal planning.

Some processed foods are going to contain fats that we want to stay away from, namely, artificial trans fats. The amount of trans fats should be indicated on the label, although I have already mentioned how "zero trans fats" can be misleading (federal guidelines allow for a "zero" reading with less than a half gram present per serving, but packaged, processed foods easily can contain more than one serving). And what foods might these be?

These can include commercial pastries and other baked goods, potato chips, fried foods, as well as frozen pizza and frozen pies. Avoiding deep-fried foods like doughnuts is a good idea. Be careful of margarine, too—the more solid it is at room temperature, the more likely it is to have higher trans fat content. Note: a number of fast-food companies claim to no longer use trans fats in cooking many of their menu items.

A good guideline here is to choose whole foods for your fat source. For dairy, choose cream, butter, and whole milk (fermented into yogurt and cheese if fresh milk is not for you)—preferably from pastured animals. Why pasture-raised? Cows grazing on pasture are part of an integrated farm system, generating farm fertility precisely where nutrients are needed—where grass is growing. True, the main dairy breeds—Holsteins, Guernseys, Jerseys—seem to still need some grain to maintain condition and keep up milk production. But grazing cows transfer nutrients to the milk: fresh grass and sunshine mean an additional bonus of some vitamins and desirable fatty acids, although maybe not as much as in fatty fish. So, the main reason to consider pasture-grazed dairy animals is because they are most likely part of a whole system: raised primarily on grass. Benefits from pasture-raised meat are similar. However, here is a good stop—think—then act moment. Think of how you feel about meat's greenhouse gas emissions, especially with meat production on a mega-scale, before you act.

Eggs are a good choice for cholesterol, as are fatty fish like salmon. Here, consider wild Pacific over caged Atlantic, as we discussed in Part 1. Plant sources of saturated fat include palm kernel oil and coconut oil. However, look for Rainforest Alliance Certified or similar "sustainable" products, since deforestation for palm oil plantations is a huge global problem. Be aware, though, that a "sustainable" label isn't a guarantee that rainforests were not cleared to grow the palm trees; but there's at least a better chance that *some* environmental standards were followed than with products that aren't labeled.

Sugars

Sugar is indeed the food that, at least in modern times, "nobody needs, but everyone craves." Gnawing sugarcane for energy and a "sugar high" is not new—most likely it's been going on for millennia. And, as I mentioned in Part 2, neither is it necessarily harmful—considering the total load of fiber all that gnawing delivers. Of course, there are other sweeteners besides sugarcane—and many of these don't have sugarcane's additional fiber. The sugar in both cane and sugar beets, for example, is disaccharide sucrose, which is absorbed from the intestines and into the bloodstream. From there, the glucose part is quickly distributed throughout the body for energy, whereas the fructose part is transported to the liver (as we discussed earlier). Sugar-sweetened beverages (soft drinks, fruit drinks, energy drinks) are the source of almost 40% of the added sugar consumed by Americans. As we saw in the work of Robert Lustig in Part 2, it's the added fructose in processed foods—especially sugary drinks—that's a problem.

There's no doubt that fructose is powerful—just a little bit can brighten our moods with the spike of dopamine it delivers. Once in the liver, fructose in high amounts is easily converted into fat—and not the good, saturated fat necessary for vital hormone production, but the excess kind around our bellies that most of us want to avoid.

Part of whole food eating is to eat fibrous plant foods, especially if we are steering away from all those convenience-food carbs. As I mentioned earlier, even sugar "in nature" comes with its own insulin-blood-spike protection, namely the fibrous part of the plant. The fiber reduces the rate of carbohydrate absorption into the intestines, and slows down the insulin response we talked about in Part 2.

Is sugar addictive? I don't know (and most other folks don't either), but we certainly seem to crave a lot of it. Robert Lustig says that we get *habituated* to it—over time, we want more and more.

So, if you're putting FoodWISE principles into practice, here's a place to start: stay away from those sugary drinks. Be especially aware of what sugar in the diet displaces: fats and fibrous carbohydrates we don't get because we're filling up on sugary carbs instead. So, sometimes the problem is not what's wrong with the food, but what *good* foods are eliminated from our diets by overconsuming processed foods. Much as mass-producers of food would like us to think otherwise, our bodies need more than just different variations on corn and soy.

Delicious Food Choices

Okay then: we've added whole foods to our list of "Do's." What else? Well, eat food that tastes good! Seek new, delicious tastes. This is what University of Florence researchers Monteleone and Dinnella from Part 2 tell us. Do not rely just on what you read or hear, but also rely on your own experience of taste, especially as you broaden your experience and learn what good food really can be. You know what a good tomato tastes like, and hopefully, a good tomato sauce.

It's important for us to keep enjoying many different food tastes—it's how we recognize quality in foods. And along the way, try to avoid the pseudoscience of diets. Diets are temporary food restriction programs that don't work as substitutes for longtime lifestyle changes of eating less sugar and more whole foods.

Making It Easy

I'll make this easy—and link it to examples of recipes at the end of the book. Bring back the fats. Cut back on carbs, especially the processed ones. Eat whole foods. It's only when we start messing with those foods—taking out the fat, adding in the preservatives, taking the "whole" out of the grains and putting in artificial vitamins instead, bringing on the sugar and salt to make up for everything we're taking away—that the food is no longer good enough.

Fats—eat a variety, but don't skimp on the saturated kind
Recipe Example: Marinated Salmon

Sweet, naturally
Recipe Example: Pear Almond Pudding

Carbohydrates—make them fibrous
Recipe Example: Vegetarian Chili

Variety of flavors and tastes
Recipe Example: Roquefort and Apple Omelet

Informed Decisions

Informed follows naturally from Whole. If you know something is a whole food, chances are you know where it came from. Or do you? How far back do you want to trace your food to determine the real cost of producing it, and, then again, how wide do you want to go to look at its impacts? There's a lot that goes into Sustainability that should be accounted for. Yet taking the time to learn whether the organic apples you're buying come from New Zealand or from the farm down the road is part of becoming an informed member of your agricultural web.

But, short of buying all your food labeled with a bar code that tells you everything involved in its production and processing, how are you going to know the history of that particular orange or package of tea? (Bar codes are actually starting to be used, for example in Europe, in tracking social and environmental impacts at the producer level and throughout the entire agricultural web.) It's hard to know whom and what you are supporting with your food purchase or restaurant meal. For your own decisions, how informed is informed enough?

Start somewhere. So, if I'm shopping, I make a mental list of what I'm ideally looking for, let's say in eggs. (Some of those considerations are discussed in Recipes in Part 4, in the section on "Eggs.") And I'm not afraid to ask questions about origin and sourcing, or the meaning of a label, at the grocery store.

For me, it's ideal to grow a lot of my food—but that's me, I like doing it—and to purchase some of the rest from trusted sources, where I know the farm operations, what the animals ate and how they were raised, and what the plants received for additional nutrients. I do, however, often default to "good enough"—for one thing, I'm just not home all the time. There are other considerations. A big one is: am I in someone else's home, on someone else's farm? Then I eat what I'm given. I make a sane, rational choice, defaulting to being sociable with the people at the dinner table and grateful for the food I'm eating. I am nevertheless delighted if there are some wholesome foods as part of the menu—well prepared, cooked, and seasoned—tastes that we don't get from many manufactured foods.

Being informed also entails stepping back and understanding how we actually make our decisions about food. We've already talked (in Part 2) about some of what goes into making food choices on a personal level. Clearly, our strong ideas and beliefs about food drive our eating behavior. Values underlie our stable, long-lasting beliefs about what is important, often forming the standards by which we live.

What's factored into our choices are our memories of good (and bad) tastes and family/childhood associations (I've shared plenty of my own throughout this book), issues we may have around body image, our tendencies toward distracted or emotional eating that might make us seek sugary foods for their "happy" neurochemical buzz—and certainly the influences of marketing. Advertising, in particular, gives us information to persuade us to buy one product over another—and it is effective. This is especially true in our nutrition-focused culture where companies make health claims for "nutrition components"—added vitamin C, added calcium, added fiber. Still, one of the biggest influences on food choice is convenience. Prepared foods dominate food buying in the United States, whether that food is a packaged meal purchased at a nearby grocery store or a pizza delivered to your door.

A big part of being informed is deciding what information you can trust. You can't decide how big a role science should play in your food choices until you know what science is saying. Of course, then again, when the sugar industry is paying for pro-sugar research, or there's bias in a study that cherry-picks favorable data, it's hard to know what information to rely on.

Use your good sense—as you think about the pro-cholesterol theories of Stephanie Seneff, or the assault on fructose of Robert Lustig, or the taste-sensory work of Erminio Monteleone and Caterina Dinnella. What did you think of Seneff's counterintuitive ideas: that cholesterol may actually have a role in changing harmful forms of sugar-damaged lipoproteins to beneficial forms? Does it make sense to you that the body squirrels away cholesterol and fat when we deprive our bodies of both? And to what end? Could degenerative diseases be explained by such dietary deficiencies? And, then, what's the take-home message for you in making your food choices? You may not be a medical researcher, but you can figure out a lot for yourself with common sense and a bit of digging around.

Again, to advance our understanding of conflicting information, we need to stop—think—then act. One question to ask is, does the advice to embrace more saturated fat fit with other information we have? It does for me, but maybe it doesn't for you—you may need more information and time to consider it. And, just maybe, Seneff's theoretical bent doesn't quite fit with how you like to get your nutrition advice. Certainly, information-gathering is a process that takes time. Reading books (like this one, I would like to think) and articles helps. But nothing works as well as experience, informed by shopping, cooking, and eating whole foods from sustainable sources, to check whether FoodWISE is right for you.

Sustainability

Sustainability is partly about what our agricultural practices are doing to the world around us. To reiterate a few problems we've looked at: the effects of chemical pesticides on other life forms (we've mentioned the case of glyphosate), uncertainties about effects of genetic engineering and other technologies on the structure of farm communities, impacts of farming practices on greenhouse gases and global climate change, and effects of subsidies and other policies and programs on farm size and farming practices.

For me, one good way to make food decisions is to try to think local "true blue" more than "global green"—even if that global food bears an "organic" sticker and the local food does not. Even if you consider just the fossil fuels used in transport and industrial-scale food manufacturing, it's easy to see why buying from overseas, or even from the other side of the United States, isn't necessarily WISE. Yet as Berners-Lee discusses for apples and bananas (among other things), long-distance shipping in itself doesn't necessarily have a big carbon impact if it is by ship—which is about 1% as much as by plane. It is clear that bigness might carry with it an economies-of-scale price advantage. Perhaps it even carries an economies-of-scale energy advantage, too—transporting many thousands of loaves of bread long distances might still add up to less fossil fuels used per loaf than, say, lower quantities more frequently transported shorter distances. But other considerations come into play, like freshness.

Or, instead of driving to the store to buy that loaf (and, admittedly, other groceries) we could be making our own (see "Gigi's Tassajara Bread Redux," in Part 4 Recipes). Or, we could subscribe to a local bread Community Supported Agriculture (CSA) if one exists, and maybe get tasty loaves delivered by bicycle to our doorstep. CSA operations sell subscriptions for delivery of food at specified intervals; they originated with small farms making weekly deliveries of fresh vegetables, but, in some communities, bakers and other food makers have adopted the business model. Add in supporting your local small-scale farmers maintaining healthy ecosystems on their land, as well as millers and bakers using locally adapted grains, and it makes "true blue" look like a good choice indeed.

Sustainable thinking isn't just about the natural environment. It also requires us to think about whether farmers themselves can be "sustained": how resilient is the social and economic agricultural web? When you're deciding what to put on your table, think about what the farmers you're buying from are doing now to ensure small farms like theirs can survive. Small- or large-scale, is the labor supply well compensated, or is lack of a well-compensated labor force a threat to the resilience of their farms?

And something else about Sustainability: Certainly, our agricultural economy for decades has enjoyed a culture of price-supported commodities—most of which are grown by large-scale farms. Further, these crops, such as corn and soy, as well as sugar beets, are prime targets for companies like Monsanto/Bayer to genetically engineer organisms that will appeal to farmers growing mass quantities of one kind of food. We've talked about possible problems with these GE crops, including pesticides used on them, and asked questions: Do the active ingredients in the pesticides appear in our corn- and soy-rich processed foods (think corn syrup and animal feeds)?

This is not an indictment of the tens of thousands of corn, soy, and sugar-beet farms and farmers. Rather, it is to say that the social consequences of price supports and genetically engineered technologies across all sizes of farms need to be looked at for unfair advantages. That just makes sense, in terms of resilience all across the board. And once we do that, keeping resilience in mind, we might have some better ideas how to support our smaller farms. (Hint: Prioritizing diversity of crops, fertility sources, and marketing channels plays a part.)

Experience-Based Thinking

Finally, there's the question of experience. Experience comes from being an active part of your agricultural web. I like to know the farmers who produce my food, and to see their farms. I like to know where the chickens are housed, to see the grass the cows are being raised on, to talk to the young person who picks the bugs off the raspberry canes.

Then again, I have personal experience with these things and so I can relate and understand somewhat. Even without that, though, I believe that information can provide secondhand—and perfectly valid—experience. We can't all be raising our own protein sources—but we can be cooking them (more on that later) and that's more likely the FoodWISE experience you'll have. Information comes in many forms—like stories. I like to gain food experiences through the stories of my friends: Why is this a favorite food? What brought them to this particular recipe?

My idea of experience includes cooking. Cooking can be boiling the water, stirring the beans, or peeling the potatoes you dug up that morning or bought from the local convenience store or Costco. And, at the end of the day, sitting down to a meal—and enjoying the tastes, no matter how simple or familiar—with the people you love.

The more we cook, trying new foods and fine-tuning the ones we know, the better we know what we are looking for in a food—which is part of our understanding of its quality. What is high quality for me may be different than what is high quality for you. For me, appearance and texture contribute to quality. Taste and aroma are important: Together, they make up flavor. The production and processing of the foods also contribute to quality. Of course, high-quality foods also should be free from pathogenic bacteria; clearly, sanitation is one criterion for quality.

Taste and aroma, for me, are crucial factors in choosing, say, one cheese over another. I vote for cheese that was made in seasoned wooden vats, because the vats affect the quality of each cheese (the aging, too, helps in producing a unique taste and aroma profile)—similar to oak barrels imparting flavor to wine.

It all sounds good. It is good. For the rest of Part 3 we'll talk about how to get to FoodWISE. You'll become a little more informed. Hopefully you'll also get inspired. In Part 4, I include some recipes to help get you cooking.

FOODWISE COOKING

Cooking is one of the most radical things we can do—especially given the huge time-saving appeal of prepared foods. Many convenient foods masquerade as Whole—like breads and wraps that have never undergone a real yeast fermentation, crunchy vegetable chips, and sweet carb- and protein-loaded bars of all sorts. More of these become available every day. Prepackaged foods are often more costly than bulk purchases—but many consumers are happy to pay for the convenience. Certainly, it takes time and energy to shop and cook.

As I advocate getting back to the kitchen, I also want to be clear that I don't suggest cooking become a chore or strictly a woman's task. This is not a call for all of us to become the rosy-cheeked housewives of my mother's generation (or the more realistic image I remember of my weary mom in one of her many aprons). That isn't what I see in the mirror. You probably don't either. And that's a good thing—we've made significant progress in the United States in improving gender roles and equity. Bringing *everyone* back into the cooking process can only further that goal. I very much like the diversity of cooks I see in my classes, and I see a lot of FoodWISE choices in their cooking.

That said, I've never seen my own shopping and cooking and growing and planting as a burden, probably because it's my passion. My mother, like many matriarchs of her generation, surely did see it as a burden—all those nice Italian meals really took their toll. Her delicious tomato sauce took two days to prepare; the gnocchi, all day. I wanted to cook like she did, which turned out to be more difficult than I thought. I watched her cook Yorkshire puddings and homemade pasta and cannoli, egg frittatas and fried cauliflower, soups and stews, donuts after school, and lemon meringue pie with lemons from our own tree. Tellingly, it's mostly the egg frittatas and fried cauliflower and stocks—the easier things—that have stuck with me (see Part 4 Recipes).

What I retained from my parents was my interest in hearty, sociable meals. So, cooking during college became a quick route to entertaining, tapping into other cultures, patronizing open-air markets. But it wasn't the utterly slow, painstaking cooking of my mother. I idolized Frances Moore Lappé, author of *Diet for a Small Planet,* while I was in graduate school—and once even got to cook dinner for her in my tiny studio apartment. I made her one of my favorite pressure cooker meals, which invariably consisted of my canned tomatoes, barley, butter, cheese, cabbage and leafy greens, and plenty of seasonings (see "Pressure Cooker Vegetable Stew," in Part 4 Recipes).

Whole, sustainable, inexpensive—my mantra also in graduate school, where I managed to subsist on twenty-two small loaves of bread a week, a bit of pasta and egg, and homemade yogurt. In one of my subsequent faculty jobs, I hosted dinners every weekend for three months to get to know my coworkers. I served virtually the same meal of salmon and potatoes and greens each time.

Cooking with an eye to time and money is what we all have to do—especially those of us with families, other caregiving responsibilities, out-of-home work, and/or limited budgets. The example comes to mind of a good friend, who manages to feed a family of eight each day—that's twenty-four individual meals; her cooking includes pureeing canned peaches as a barely sweet sauce for some high-fiber pancakes, cutting apples to serve with peanut butter, and poaching wild salmon bought in quantity at Costco for dinner (not all in the same meal, of course). She uses some "easy" items like canned tuna for lunch and then adds a few of my home-canned dilly beans chopped up for good measure and flavor. Easy meals—cooked with love, quick to prepare, a mix of convenience and budget ingenuity.

I want to say, too, that if you know how to cook only a few meals, or feel comfortable handling only basic foods like rice, chicken, potatoes, there is a lot of variety you can enjoy—even if you're on a tight budget. Many of the recipes in Part 4 are for the budget-conscious—for example, using eggs and vegetables in soups, curries, and chili.

Variety was one of the main messages of back-to-basics cooking pioneer M. F. K. Fisher. One of her most well-known books, *How to Cook a Wolf*, dates from World War II. It is full of creative recipes for soups, fish, eggs, bread, and beef—all on a budget. Pasta water becomes soup stock, feed-store grains become your breakfast cereal, egg-boiling becomes more art than science by varying the "boiling minutes" (and thus egg texture) giving you almost a new food each time you cook. Our tastes *and* needs can bring us to a wonderful focus on food basics and economics.

Tamar Adler also gives us this no-nonsense approach in her *An Everlasting Meal: Cooking with Economy and Grace.* Cooking with economy and grace means getting every ounce of juice and gristle from meats, every micronutrient from a vegetable. Other cookbook authors also talk about eking out nutrients from odd foods and microbes—all good advice, and very doable. Clearly, taking the time to cook at home and rediscover simple ingredients is possible on a budget. Read, and explore.

So, to begin, let's go shopping.

FOODWISE SHOPPING

Let's go back to the supermarket now, bringing the ideas of FoodWISE with us. We'll be looking for Whole foods with Sustainable production, about which we're well-Informed, foods that either build on Experiences we've had or offer us something new. Of course, if we're going to shop informed, it helps to go in knowing our "ideal," "good enough," and "in a pinch."

Start with a shopping list so you won't walk away with a bunch of quick impulse buys—açai-flavored xylitol-sweetened chewing gum, or barbeque-flavored potato chips you never intended to buy anyway. Shop mainly on the outside of the store in the produce, dairy, and meat sections; avoid those aisles of processed foods in the middle.

Make a list, asking yourself simple questions. And don't worry: this gets easier. Soon, shopping FoodWISE should feel pretty automatic. At least, it's gotten that way for me; it's second nature now to walk through the grocery store, asking...

Is it Whole? That's pretty straightforward, and should make shopping fast. Try to avoid the processed stuff.

Am I Informed? Do I know where the food comes from? Does the food have some saturated fat? Does this "organic" label actually mean a smaller carbon footprint? Can I tell? Does it matter?

Is it Sustainable? Here, again, comes the question of "organic." As we saw in Part 1, "organic" isn't always the best option. The Environmental Working Group's famous "Dirty Dozen" list is helpful in terms of figuring out what produce you should prioritize to buy organic—which foods, if farmed conventionally, involve the most harmful growing practices—and which don't. I buy organic strawberries, spinach, and apples, but when it comes to avocados I have to stop—think—then act. Avocados are not on the "dirty" list—in fact, they're on the Working Group's "clean list," because such a small amount of chemicals are used to grow these tough-skinned fruits. But, I still want to know where they are coming from—if from Mexico's Michoacán state where investigative journalism reports have raised questions about deforestation and pesticide poisonings, then I might look for an organic label or other certification.

What is my Experience with this food? Do I have personal experience with where it came from or how it was processed, and therefore can form my own views about how FoodWISE it is? What's my experience with the brand of this food? Do I trust it? What's my experience with preparing and cooking this food, do I know how to do it? Maybe the answer is "no," but you feel like trying it anyway—maybe a friend recommended it, or maybe you just feel adventurous.

At the risk of stating the obvious, also look for food you know you'll actually use. How much do you need to buy for just one or two meals? If you're eating meat, consider getting less than you would buy normally but of a higher quality—for example, pasture-raised. Whole chicken is usually a good economical bet, but I choose local (and pastured) over "natural," which refers mostly to a lack of antibiotics. I also want to know the source of the chicken: I don't want to buy meat produced on massive farms far away. Neither do I spend my precious pennies on FoodWISE chicken every week. I buy less, but pastured (or we raise our own—but that's not every year). I buy preserved meats (salami, prosciutto, pastrami, ham) only occasionally, and mostly when I'm entertaining. I vary my protein sources with kidney beans and garbanzo beans.

Milk, to me, is easy. I look for a bottle of Grade A fresh, raw milk. Others might turn to Twin Brook Creamery's non-homogenized low-temperature vat-pasteurized Jersey milk, which comes from right in our own county (see story in Part 1). If you don't have milk that is so obviously good in your locale, check out the processors and distributors that sell milk in your stores. For example, one of ours, Darigold, does not carry milk from cows raised with recombinant bovine growth hormone.

So … here's my master shopping list. What I actually end up buying— and how much of it—depends not only on what I find in the store, but also on what I have in mind for a meal: am I entertaining, do I feel like experimenting with something new? Consider making some of these foods your staples, buy in bulk, and you can fill your cart in a very FoodWISE way.

My FoodWISE shopping list

Usually, I get just a few items from each category. I consider FoodWISE guidelines, and sometimes grow or produce items myself. For anything that is not local (almonds, coffee, chocolate, to name a few), I look for sustainable growing practices or a certification to that effect.

DAIRY

Butter

Cheese

Milk

Yogurt

OTHER FAT AND PROTEIN

Chicken

Dried beans (black, garbanzo, kidney, lentils, split peas)

Eggs

Fish (usually local salmon)

Ground beef

Nut butter (cashew, almond, peanut)

Pork

Tofu

GRAINS

Barley, millet

Brown rice

Steel-cut oats

Wheat flour (I actually don't bake much bread these days; if I do, I go for the coarsest whole wheat flour I can find, or mill my own, and add whole foods like corn or wheat berries [but be sure to soak these—I had a FoodWISE experience once by not soaking the rock-hard berries before adding them to the beautiful bread dough I had carefully made; the dough was ruined])

NUTS AND SEEDS

Almonds

Cashews

Pecans

Pistachios

Walnuts

Chia seeds

Flaxseeds

Sesame seeds

Sunflower seeds

FRUIT

Year round:

   Apples (fresh or from cold storage)

   Bananas

Seasonal (some from my yard):

Blueberries

Cherries

Figs

Pears

Plums

Strawberries

SPICES AND HERBS

(some of which I have in my garden)

(I buy organic spices, to avoid irradiation processing)

Basil

Black pepper (also white)

Chili powder

Cinnamon

Ginger

Lavender

Mint

Oregano

Paprika

Parsley

Red pepper, crushed or flakes

Rosemary

Tarragon

Thyme

Sage

Sea salt

Summer savory

Vanilla

VEGETABLES

Broccoli

Carrots

Cauliflower

Celery

Corn

Cucumbers

Eggplants

Green beans

Lettuce

Mushrooms

Onions

Peppers

Potatoes

Spinach

Squash

Sweet potatoes

Tomatoes

CONDIMENTS, OILS

Coconut oil

Extra virgin olive oil

Tahini (a sesame-seed paste)

Tamari (a form of fermented soy)

Worcestershire sauce (challenging to find as a whole food; look for low-sugar)

CANNED OR BOTTLED GOODS

Beans (black, garbanzo, kidney, lentils)

Capers

Diced or whole chili peppers

Hot pepper sauce

Mustards (Dijon, whole grain and other coarse mustards)

Olives

Peas

Salsa

Tomatoes (crushed, diced, paste, whole peeled)

Tuna or salmon

Vinegars (balsamic, cider, red wine, white)

BEVERAGES
Coffee

Teas

What's notable is what's *not* on the list: croissants and bagels, biscuits and cereal, granola bars, noodles, rolls and breads, chips and dips, fish sticks, hot dogs. Some of these are foods I *do* eat, on occasion—but usually when I am out and about, and they may not be my first choice. If I do eat them, I try to consider their source. I usually don't buy pasta because I prefer less-processed whole grains or vegetables—which are delightful with the same sauces I would normally add to the pasta. Otherwise, my list is straightforward, and it's what I like to cook with—mostly whole foods.

The time I spend cooking is one of the best parts of my day. It's a strong statement about how I value my time. Even just opening a can of vegetables and adding some herbs is cooking in my view. It's a clear and blunt declaration that the time spent preparing food is important, as is the time spent shopping or gathering food.

I believe that the time and energy it takes to shop and cook are a critical part of experiencing the agricultural web. Cooking is the final step, the opportunity to put all that you know and appreciate about Whole foods and Whole farming into the food you eat. Whether you cook for your family of eight or your family of one, rediscovering whole and simple ingredients, and experimenting with them in new and exciting ways, is key to becoming FoodWISE.

FOODWISE EATING OUT

Being FoodWISE is about learning for ourselves what foods work best for our minds and bodies, budgets, and schedules. Everyone can do FoodWISE.

Not everybody can grow a lot of their own food or buy fresh fruit and vegetables at their local co-op. Some of us aren't going to get very far in the kitchen—maybe we don't even have one. Maybe we work long hours and just don't have the energy at the end of the day (or night). Maybe some of us are residential dormitory students with limited cooking options. Maybe cooking for oneself just isn't as much fun. I must admit that while writing this food book, ironically most of my FoodWISE experience was limited to "cooking" coffee, boiling eggs, making cheese, and adding salad dressing (not my own) to fresh garden salads from my local food co-op.

Finding the time to both cook and eat can be challenging. I get that. For a variety of reasons, we eat out. Some of us eat out a lot. Well, here's the FoodWISE override: Look out for your own welfare, making choices that support your personal and informed view of food. Still, when we're eating out in restaurants, waiting in line at the food truck, or browsing the glass case at the supermarket deli—how do we deploy Whole, Informed, Sustainable, Experience-based thinking?

It is challenging to stay FoodWISE when eating out, although not impossible. For one thing, a FoodWISE approach does not mean being fussy or rigid. Whether at a restaurant or convenience store, we should consider ourselves doing well if we choose Whole *or* Informed *or* Sustainable *or* Experience.

With travel, or dealing with short lunch hours or long work meetings, sometimes we don't plan very well what we are going to eat. We may be at the mercy of the hot dog stand or downstairs café or corner tapas bar. Even in these situations, we can prioritize some whole food.

At the hot dog stand, I might ditch the white bread, slather on the sauerkraut, and spoon up the relish (especially if it's not too sugary). Pickles? Sure. Or I might keep the bun and heap some butter on it (if it's real butter).

What about hamburgers and fries? How do I feel—considering our shared world—about greenhouse gas emissions from the beef feedlots supplying the meat for the hamburger? Or the subsidies for the corn and soybean oils for animal feed, or the antibiotics and hormones used in industrial-scale meat production? I know that fries are made less and less with hydrogenated vegetable oils, but a lot of pesticides are used on industrial-scale potatoes and they're on the Environmental Working Group's "Shopper's Guide" to the "Dirty Dozen" pesticide-contaminated produce. Well, that meal is not WISE, but if I eat it, at least I'm informed.

On the other hand, I might choose instead a salad with oil and vinegar. Or, I might go ahead and chow down on the burger, source be damned (for now), and try to find some vegetables to go with it. I might not be contributing right then to a FoodWISE economy, but I am doing the best I can. Is this "good enough"? Probably—and I'll be on the lookout for something other than another big burger for my next meal.

Sustainable fish, as we saw in Part 1, is challenging. With some exceptions (e.g., Pacific salmon, freshwater fish elsewhere), overfishing (think some species of tuna, or Chilean sea bass), and pollution and toxicity (think farmed shellfish from certain countries) can be serious problems. So I want to be very selective when ordering it out.

We tend to think of beef, pork, chicken, fish, and other meat as being the protein in a main course, but really there are lots of other plant-based options. Eating out for me includes a lot of plant-based soups, salads, and stir-fries. And if I can find them for a good price at a good restaurant, all the better. Vegetables, though, can be expensive no matter where you are eating out. Cosmetic (no blemishes!) and freshness standards add enormously to the cost of vegetables.

When I eat out, I look for something I rarely make at home—something that's maybe just a little beyond my threshold of time or skill. I know that eating whole food invariably means a good marriage of tastes that often makes the dish exquisite—maybe a beautifully clear consommé. I've had delicious soups and stir-fries, vegetable chilis and salads, or vegetable curries and chutneys—all in restaurants.

I am fearless about splitting dishes. I try as many as I can at a meal, sharing with a friend so we can both sample widely. I am careful with restaurant bread—usually it's the commercial, industrial-scale type with a chemical fermentation at best, and I avoid it.

But restaurants aren't meant to be survived; they are meant to be enjoyed. I do believe in a democracy of tastes and choices, and there is no shame in settling for "good enough" occasionally. For me, that means being informed, and choosing as whole a food as possible, and certainly a tasty one. That's what we need to do sometimes to get by in a world inundated with convenience foods—and, oftentimes, little choice.

I freely admit that understanding and appreciating FoodWISE principles is easier than continuing to live by them day after day. But that's just it. FoodWISE is taking one day at a time. I myself address the challenge of FoodWISE every day. Getting wiser in our food choices is how we're going to change our shared world to one that's more Whole and Sustainable.

But there's also good enough. Thirty percent FoodWISE over a whole day? A whole month? What about just sometimes? Or just when we're eating at home? Are there some situations where it makes sense to choose Sane over Sustainable? When we're eating out? With friends?

Well, yes—and the example I think of is the take-away lesson from the women's self-defense class I once completed: *Just run!* In the six-week-long course, I learned lots of moves. At the end I asked: If someone is coming at me, which move do I use, how do I decide? Which one is the most effective? The instructor's response: Just run. But, I said, I took this class, so many weeks—and all I'm supposed to do is *run?*

Clearly, the instructor thought that was the best fallback option. And even though I had learned a lot, the instructor knew that it wasn't enough for me to get by in every possible situation. Sometimes you just can't figure stuff out and you have to make do. When you have more time, maybe, it's easier to think things through. But, for a meal on a busy night when you have a paper due the next day or a birthday party to plan or your in-laws are coming to town, you're going to have to settle for good enough.

So, with FoodWISE: you've learned some guidelines. I hope you can follow them. I believe it is possible to live a FoodWISE life. At least try, because that is where we need to be. If everyone is trying, much of the time, then we are going to get there.

MY FOODWISE

Nothing is simple. FoodWISE is not just about your body; it's also about your brain and your emotions, making decisions about foods that nourish you. But it also includes experience about the shared world that we are a part of. That experience makes me more empathetic—to celebrate the innovation of some of our bigger farmers trying to do the right thing, as well as the diligence of the small farmers.

Empathy allows me to, at least in part, see the world as others do—and keeps me from getting too smug and preachy. In this shared worldview, advocating for resilience includes, for example, pushing for changes in toxic farm working conditions (exposure to pesticides, long hours, backbreaking work). This makes me interested in worker advocacy groups, but also in dining clubs, CSAs, food networks, trade reform groups, and seed-saving organizations.

Our personal choices can't take on the world's food problems single-handedly. But by living as FoodWISE as we can, maybe we can start to push toward a more Sustainable future. And that's going to mean buying in (literally) to organizations and movements that support needed food reform at all levels.

I am convinced that large-scale farms need to be more resilient, with the right incentives to make that happen, and that small-scale integrated farms need to be more financially solvent—holding both accountable to Sustainability. To me, the following would comprise my ideal foodshed:

Traceable—so we know where our food comes from. Part of this is accurate labeling for foods that are genetically engineered or produced with—for example, glyphosate; but also, knowing what's locally produced. Even better is being able to visit the farm and field to see, smell, taste, and understand the roots of our food. This also means restricting cheap goods coming from inequitable food production systems in other states and in other countries.

Regenerative—with foods from systems that are more closed-loop and integrated. This means that most of the fertility is generated on the farm, whether from livestock or cover crops. I prefer "organic" because I know better what's in it (for animals, somewhere, somehow, there's pasture, and grass and animals managed in rotational grazing) and what's not (antibiotics, genetically engineered organisms, municipal sewage sludge). Although I've criticized "Big Organic," I nevertheless remain grateful for the organic label. For one thing, the lack of pesticides is a big deal. But organic could be so much better. I want to support addressing some of organic's biggest challenges, including the technical needs and financing to develop organically bred seeds; and, better support of the local, integrated farming that organic farming can be. A case in point is just a dozen miles from where I live: Viva Farms—committed to supporting 100% small-grower organic agriculture and providing both resources and skills to make it happen. Viva Farms is doing its bit to change the face of farming in my part of the United States— more women farmers and more Hispanic farmers.

Humane—with high standards for confinement operations and mass long-distance transporting of live animals. I also would scrutinize processing facilities, and all big industrial-scale operations involving animals.

Focused on revaluing tastes and biodiversity—maintaining a diverse variety of plants and animals, which means protecting the breeds of livestock and varieties of seeds that are the foundation of agricultural biodiversity.

Focused on revaluing quality—emphasizing flavor, loosening rigid ideas about appearance (size, shape), and favoring the absence of chemical contaminants or adulterants. Certainly the ability to recognize quality increases as we experiment more with food tastes and those memories become stronger.

Focused on revaluing cooking and convivial eating—eating for happiness, that is, nourishing our bodies with healthy food, while simultaneously making food choices that economically and environmentally support the communities in which we live. This involves Whole-food meals with friends and family, as well as dining in community. (For me, my community is often student-centered; I do a lot of eating with my students.)

Characterized by access, resilience, and reducing vulnerability—ensuring widespread access to good food—both growing and eating it. We need to dramatically reduce food security vulnerabilities that are tied to race, income, age, and gender. Food insecurity is more than the absence of a grocery store in an urban neighborhood that creates a food desert. We need to work to end systematic marginalization of many people in our country, and work for effective government intervention.

And so, what is your vision for the future of food in your life? In your community? Whatever you believe, now is the moment to stop—think— then act. Act with compassion for yourselves and empathy for others, and, if it helps, take FoodWISE with you along the way.

OUR FOODWISE: INTERESTS AND EMPATHY

As we talked about in the Introduction, experience leads to empathy—the ability to understand and have compassion for other living beings—and empathy results in better decisions about food. But in talking about empathy, we also should be talking about the common interests we all have: being free from illness and disease; having adequate resources for a long, healthy life; being free from racism, discrimination, and marginalization of all forms. So those common interests are where we should start on our collective FoodWISE journey.

Our food choices (which is what FoodWISE is about) are partly shaped by our beliefs. We've looked at where beliefs come from; we each have our own, different from each other's; none are more wrong or more right. But, inevitably, there are better and worse ways to realize those common interests. One of the better ways is to use science, because science describes the real world we live in and provides us with the kind of information we need to make realistic food choices. If we're not dealing with real scientific knowledge, then we're not going to take actions that have the desired outcomes in the real world. We're not going to be well, and we're not going to maintain small integrated family farms, and we're not going to avoid climate change.

But first, we have to get everyone agreeing on the interests: healthy us, healthy world. Then, get everyone understanding where our ideas on what to do to achieve those interests come from (including how our beliefs are formed). Then—ideally—get everyone agreeing that sound science should be a main basis for deciding on actions. That could be difficult for some to accept—because beliefs sometimes have been shaped by deceptive arguments more than values. But also, we need to accept that values do play a role in deciding some things—for example, whether to eat meat or not—and that differing values are valid and have to be acknowledged.

I explain some of my own values and where they come from in the stories woven through the book: I like tomatoes, I like milking sheep, I like most any farms that are smaller than mega-sized. You don't have to. But those values of mine help explain my views of other things I talk about in this book. And if you empathize with me, you'll understand what I'm getting at, and it may push you along on your own journey.

In addition, empathy is personally rewarding, by giving us a better understanding and view of our complicated world, and leading us to try new things and have a richer life. Clearly, empathizing with each other is key to a successful FoodWISE journey.

WE NEED: TO BE FOODWISE AND CHOOSE EXPERIENCE

In Part 4, I want to share my FoodWISE journey in recipes. So far, I've been doing a lot of Informing—I know! We've looked at Sustainability, and thought a lot about Whole foods. But FoodWISE is all about getting out there and learning for yourself—learning what tastes good, learning what feels right for you. It's about Experiencing food firsthand. So I've included these recipes—foods I have made a part of my life, foods I've learned about from family and friends and students, foods that have meant something to me in my FoodWISE journey. With each recipe, you'll have the chance to see what makes it FoodWISE. And since Experience-based thinking is so key to everything I believe in, I've included some stories as well—my experiences—and what these recipes mean to me, or to the wider agricultural web.

So settle into your kitchen, or your favorite reading nook, or a table at your local market café. Take a look at these recipes. Pick up or harvest some whole food ingredients—and don't forget to experiment along the way.

PART 4

WISE Stories to Share: The Recipes

Before you get started with these recipes, here are some general notes to keep in mind. Further comments can be found at https://wp.wwu.edu /gigiberardi/category/foodwise-resilient-farms-and-nourishing-foods-blog.

LET'S GET COOKING (SOME GENERAL NOTES TO KEEP IN MIND)

Preparation time and utensils. Recipes with fresh vegetables may require considerable time to prepare, wash, and cut the veggies, so the times I give are approximate. They depend on many things, including how much washing your veggies need and how quick you are with a knife—and what kind of knives you have. (Where I lived in Switzerland, we had a dozen knives for different vegetables, and different *parts* of vegetables; back home, honestly, sometimes I make do with a regular dinner knife.) Dry beans also need to be cleaned and washed, then soaked and simmered. If you can get all the ingredients ready—*mise en place*—this will aid enormously in increasing your efficiency in the kitchen. Importantly, "Prep time" usually refers to *both the preparation and cooking times* together. I note also if you will need some unusual utensils.

Preciseness, weighing, and measuring. Most quantities, including solid ingredients, are given in volumes—¼ cup flour—not weights—30 g. This is not as precise but more realistic for how people think of quantities. However, some ingredients that are packaged or sold by weight—like an 8-oz container of yogurt, or one pound of almonds—are listed as such.

Batch size. I like cooking, but I *love* leftovers. I like to make BIG batches. I've tried to rein in this practice a bit here, and warn you about the size of batches (for example, the "Roasted Vegetables" recipe makes two sheets-full, the bread recipe produces multiple loaves). But, you'll need to be on the lookout, too, for recipes you might want to cut in half.

Yields and number of servings. These are approximate. The number of servings will depend on serving size and what else you serve with the dish.

Techniques and equipment. I rarely explain cooking techniques—mincing, dicing, or slicing, but sometimes explain equipment.

FoodWISE. As I said in the FoodWISE shopping section, I try to source my food with FoodWISE guidelines, sometimes growing and producing the item myself. But empathy in the food system suggests compassion, too, for yourself first as a shopper, as a cook, and as the final consumer—you're just going to do the best you can to find Whole foods from Whole farms.

A few comments on ingredients:

Salt and black pepper. Table salt is typically mined and processed, with at least a dozen allowable additives. Sea salt, however, usually goes through an evaporation process that leaves some trace minerals. So, is sea salt the Food-WISE choice? Taste for yourself and see if there is a difference. For me, there is! The sea salts tend to be more flavorful, and have a rougher texture—I use less. For all of us, FoodWISE means making these decisions given your own resources and experience. I prefer, and use, fresh-ground sea salt and black pepper for all the recipes included here, but for simplicity and clarity I've simply used the terms "salt" and "black pepper."

Water. Use filtered water if you think you need to. I tend to use filtered water for anything requiring fermentation, to avoid any chlorine residual from municipal water supplies.

Non-local foods, convenience foods. I use them. Take a look at the spice powders in the "Vegetarian Curry" recipe (for example, cinnamon and ginger)—I don't prepare them myself. There are some whole foods I could actually get fresh, then dry, then pound with a pestle and mortar—but I don't. There are some that would require so much additional work on my part that it is unrealistic to expect that I grow, make, or process them myself. As I said earlier, "More whole, yes? But that's a time-consuming process I have not yet embraced." Additionally, there are some foods in these recipes that I cannot get fresh locally (almonds, citrus, coffee, and chocolate, to name a few). Yes, we have local companies that make chocolate products as well as local coffee roasters—but their ingredients aren't local. I do tend to buy coffee and chocolate with labels certifying sustainability and/or fair labor practices. Once again, non-local foods are difficult to avoid (but, as has been pointed out, they don't necessarily have the largest carbon footprint either). The important takeaway is to approach purchasing non-local or convenience foods in a way that is as FoodWISE as possible.

Energy use. Take a look at the "Crispy Almonds" recipe. What about setting the oven on 200 degrees all night to dehydrate a pound of nuts? There's an energy cost there, and maybe using a more renewable energy resource like solar drying fits more with your view of carbon footprint and energy use.

***

Now, let's get cooking.

EGGS

Eggs come from some of the easiest livestock to keep, and now with the availability of "pasture-raised" or "cage-free" or "organic and no antibiotics" in the stores, you're all set. We've already discussed how natural chicken behavior doesn't happen in crowded, 50,000- or even 5,000-chicken confinement laying operations. If you buy your eggs, please spend your pennies on free-ranging birds!

Of course, there are zero-mile eggs: those produced in your own backyard. Be aware: with the occasional truant dog and marauding owl, we've found that keeping small backyard livestock like ducks, rabbits, and chickens can be challenging even in our quiet town of Bellingham.

The transformation of habitat and chicken feed to a human food high in cholesterol and protein is amazing to me. Free-ranging chickens are eating plants and animals in their natural environment, although they don't eat a whole lot—for grass, just the tips of the blades. The scorched-earth policy they seem to execute in your yard comes from their scratching around for seeds, earthworms, and slugs; and also for the scraps of food you give them: voilà, in situ compost—composting of the scraps they didn't eat, right in or on the ground.

There's so much about eggs that is FoodWISE: their expense is manageable, and they're a whole food that comes with its own packaging. I experiment a lot with eggs: adding avocado and other fats like coconut to my omelets and frittatas, and adding all sorts of vegetables, cooked and uncooked. You'll see in the recipes that I use butter for the fat—butter that is strong and firm and whole. It's not softened with feisty industrial hydrogen. The slightly nutty smell brings back the butter-rich omelets of my childhood. Should the butter be salted or unsalted? Most people enjoy the taste of salt, especially in eggs, breads, and tomato dishes. I almost always use salted butter, but try for yourself. Lard, which I've cooked with some, does not seem to have a smell, but when cut with coconut oil smells sweet. Keep in mind that using a lot of cheese can overwhelm the other ingredients in an egg dish. Don't get me wrong: I make it, I love it. But that omelet made with a cup of cheese is going to taste like, well, cheese. Which might be exactly the taste you want. But if it is not—use sparingly.

Vegetable Scramble

Serves 4

Equipment: Medium-sized frying pan or cast-iron skillet, a spatula (a scraper or flipper, like what you would use for pancakes), and a small mixing bowl

Prep time: About 15 minutes

INGREDIENTS

2 large garlic cloves, peeled and minced (I avoid crushing the tender bulb; I find the dish more flavorful when I haven't pressed, squashed, or squeezed the garlic, but gently sliced it into smaller pieces)

½ onion (yellow or red), diced into small cubes

1 medium-sized carrot, thinly sliced to about ¼-inch thickness

1½ green peppers, diced

6 eggs, whisked

1 tbsp butter, for cooking

⅛ tsp each salt and black pepper, or to taste

Optional: Garnishes such as washed spinach leaves, edible flowers (like calendula), sprigs of herbs (rosemary, sage), pieces of cut fruit like apple or pear

PREPARATION

Wash or rinse the vegetables, and cut as noted (or into whatever different sizes you'd like to see in your scramble). The idea is to cut vegetables in sizes so that they will cook at about the same time: dense carrots take longer to cook (so slice thinner) than lighter, moister green peppers.

Prepare the eggs just before adding them to the pan. I figure on about 1½ eggs per person. Using a small mixing bowl, gently tap the egg on the edge of the bowl. Find a crack, pry it open a bit, and empty into the bowl. *Plop!* Inspect the yolk—a firm, bright yolk indicates a fresh egg, but also something about the chicken's feed. (Plant pigments contribute to the orangeness of the yolk; even the type of grain can affect the color—with wheat and barley making a lighter yolk.) Whisk the eggs (tilt the bowl slightly and quickly stir) with a fork or small whisk. (I love whisking and have three or four different sizes of whisks—from yard sales and secondhand markets.) Whisking for a good minute or so adds air to the eggs, and makes for a somewhat fluffier dish.

Heat butter in a medium-sized frying pan (I use a cast-iron skillet) on medium heat.

Add the garlic; cook gently, stirring occasionally until softened (not to the point of scorching!). The garlic should change color, darkening a bit.

Then, add onions, cooking enough to soften.

Add the sliced carrot. After a few minutes, add the green pepper. Don't overcook; you want good texture, not mush. The green pepper and carrot—latecomers to the melee—should have a slight crunch.

Add the egg mixture, letting it spread luxuriously to the edges of the pan. It helps to tilt the pan, until the mixture starts to curl up the sides. You want to quickly but thoroughly heat the mixture. Gently scrape or lift the mixture off the bottom of the pan (until you see the eggs solidifying), scooping up the partially cooked vegetables and softening the egg curds. I like my eggs on the dry side. How do you like yours? A little jiggly, or firm? It's up to you; the longer you gently move the mixture around, the more firmly it will set.

Toward the end of cooking, add a shake or two of salt and black pepper (I use a shaker with a grinder so it's freshly ground).

Roughly divide the scramble into four pieces and, using a spatula, loosen the side and bottom of each piece and lift onto plates. Serve with some garnish on each: washed spinach leaves, edible flowers (like the pretty yellow-orange calendula), and/or sprigs of herbs (rosemary, sage). You can also serve with cut-up fruit such as apples or pears.

Roquefort and Apple Omelet

Serves 4

An omelet is a bit fancier than an egg scramble, because you fold the egg mixture around the filling in the middle. But, basically, the formula is the same: eggs mixed with something, cooked on the stove in a frying pan. Here is one favorite recipe; I like the strong cheese and fresh fruit contrast.

You can substitute any strong-tasting cheeses—I'd suggest blue cheese for this recipe, like English Stilton or Italian Gorgonzola. But, try local first! Making blues is popular among artisan cheesemakers. In my county we have Twin Sisters Creamery dedicated to the production of Whatcom Blue—delicious!

Equipment: Large-sized frying pan or cast-iron skillet and lid, especially if you are going to flip it (see preparation), a small mixing bowl, and a spatula

Prep time: About 15 minutes

INGREDIENTS

6 eggs, whisked (see "Vegetable Scramble" recipe instructions, above)

3 oz Roquefort cheese, crumbled (I use my own, it's strong and pungent) (Roquefort is a good raw-milk cheese to try; you easily can find it for sale in the United States, due in part to its unfriendly-to-microbes high salt content)

3–4 tbsp grated Parmesan or other aged cheese

1 small–medium green apple, finely sliced

1 tbsp butter, for cooking

⅛ tsp each salt and black pepper, or to taste

PREPARATION

In a small mixing bowl, mix together eggs, cheeses, and apple.

Heat butter in large-sized frying pan or cast-iron skillet on medium heat. Add mixture so it spreads quickly (you can help by tilting it) and cook until omelet is starting to get firm and pull away from the sides. You may want to tip the pan occasionally to better distribute the mixture for more even cooking.

Add salt and pepper.

Using a spatula, fold the omelet in half when it is mostly cooked (after maybe 6–8 minutes), and then cover it (for another 2–3 minutes, or until done). Some prefer to flip the entire omelet before it is completely cooked (when the edges have just begun to turn white), then adding filling and folding it over; if you want to do this, just know that timing (and practice) is everything.

Remove from heat and use a spatula to loosen omelet onto a serving plate. (See notes for garnishes under "Vegetable Scramble" recipe, above.)

DAIRY

As for cows, well, I admit I can't be objective; for me, the cow is a mystical being—including the cows at Our Lady of the Rock Monastery on Shaw Island, where I help out. At our own sheep micro-dairy (Three Sheep Creamery), we use a number of different practices, including biodynamics. Biodynamics is a form of regenerative farming: inputs are generated from the farm itself—about as close to a closed-loop, low-input, integrated farming system as is possible. In other words, you recycle and reuse everything feasible, like putting livestock manure back on the plants as fertilizer. A unique feature of this method is that it is almost homeopathic in nature: small amounts of fermented herbs enliven or vitalize composts of green wastes (grass clippings and food wastes), layered with dried hay (brown wastes) and manure from the monastery's lactating cow. The resources that are needed most are those of the farmer him/herself: strong will and a generous spirit, open to the cosmos.

Cows are big, some weighing close to 800 pounds. With my aversion to big horses, I thought I'd never be able to put myself underneath a cow. But I've milked several, and they aren't all as well behaved as the monastery's cow, Claire. Of course, Claire prefers the nuns, who milked her twice a day, day in and day out, for over six years. It would seem a no-brainer to don the same outfit when I milked; so, to imitate the nuns' blue denim work habits and white veil, I have worn a blue cotton jumper and a white milkmaid-type hat. But it's not just the clothes that make the difference—it's the touch. I've learned that touch is also hugely important in carefully handling the raw milk so as to avoid contamination. So is proper aging of cheeses—to achieve the right moisture, acidity, and salt levels to maximize flavor and safety.

At both Our Lady of the Rock monastery and its original Abbey, Regina Laudis, most cheeses are made with raw milk. At the Abbey, Sister Noella Marcellino, who started making a fungal-ripened cheese without the addition of commercial cultures in 1977, observed microbial succession on the ripening cheese in her cellar over the years. Her experience as an artisanal cheesemaker led to her doctoral research on the biodiversity of cheese-ripening fungi in traditional French caves. You can read about her in the *New Yorker's* "Raw Faith" article, and see her in action in a Harvard public lecture series. She's also featured in Michael Pollan's book *Cooked*. At the Shaw Island monastery, Mother Thérèse, the prioress, has been making cheese for at least as long.

Cheese

Milk wants to be cheese—it begins to sour soon after it leaves the udder unless you refrigerate it. This makes cheese a kind of naturally processed food. Of course, supermarket cheese is a little bit different: chemicals are added and the rigorous pasteurization and other manufacturing required in factory-produced cheese does a lot to standardize it, but also to eliminate certain flavors you can get with homemade or artisanal cheese. If you're Informed, though, you know that whole milk is full of fats and proteins (it's the protein plus glue-like calcium that helps hold the cheese together, while fats provide texture, flavor, and aroma), while being very low in carbohydrates. Experiment and experience: cheese can be a bit like wine—no two "vintages" are exactly the same. It's worth trying as many producers's cheeses as you can.

I have become a cheesemaker. In the past, I've milked cows, sheep, and goats—and now raise sheep. I am devoted to my sheep and their rich milk, so high in fat that you can freeze it and it changes little in quality. But there's something extraordinary about the taste of fresh goat milk cheese, too—otherwise known as chèvre. I add a bit of culture and coagulant to fresh goat milk, and then let the forming curd shed all its whey. I scoop the wet curd, still clinging to its own expressed whey, from the pot on the stove onto the cloth that I hang from a kitchen cabinet knob. Fast forward 8–12 hours later. The curd is dry now, so you can peel the cloth away: it's solid chèvre. I lightly salt it, and find that first bite to be a burst of strong earthiness, a feisty ruminant's (I still have scars from the goats' kicking) contribution to whole food gastronomy.

The easiest cheeses to make are the soft cheeses; the harder are ... well, not for the faint of heart, if for no other reason than they are messy. Two gallons of cow milk slims down to two pounds of solid cheese, and that liquid needs to drain somewhere. For a while, it was into too-small pots and ultimately onto my kitchen floor.

The recipes for cheesemaking are simple—and eerily similar. You warm milk (and maybe add microbial cultures), add a coagulator (usually rennet of some sort); then, after a half hour or so, cut the solidified curd that has separated from the whey. Some cheeses require more cooking at this point. Eventually, the drained solids are pressed into rounds (or squares or triangles)—but don't forget the whey.

At the right acidity, and the right temperature, you can recapture even more solids from the whey—but, oh, how this simple procedure defeats even the best of my cheesemaking students (and sometimes practitioners) so that sometimes only a pale smear of milk solids results from the heating. But, if you do heat the whey correctly (hint: almost immediately after draining off the cheese curds), your reward is handfuls of beautiful, fresh ricotta. A lot of cheesemaking means a lot of ricotta. And there are many things you can do with the ricotta.

One of my favorite uses for it is making a cheesecake with a simple recipe from *Joy of Cooking*. Or, you can take the smooth and creamy cheese and make a wonderful spread with dried fruit and nuts, or make it more savory, with herbs and pepper. Or, with a few eggs, a little olive oil, and a lot of finely chopped herbs (thyme, rosemary, tarragon, marjoram), you can bake a little soufflé in about a half hour at 350 degrees. The result is a massive amount of delicious food—all with one pound of ricotta.

Easy and Wholesome Cream Cheese

(ADAPTED FROM SALLY FALLON'S *NOURISHING TRADITIONS*)
Yield: 2 cups whey and 2 cups cream cheese

Separating milk into curds and whey is doubly delicious. Whey is a terrific starter culture for lacto-fermented vegetables (like in kimchi), or for soaking grains or nuts as for "Crispy Almonds" (recipe below). The soft cream cheese produced is delicious, and if you let it sit for several days, it just ferments that much longer, adding to its beneficial bacteria (and pungent fragrance) load.

I prefer fresh milk. I'm fortunate to have my own dairy animals, although there's part of the year when they aren't producing milk. If you're not quite ready to start keeping dairy animals, you can likely purchase raw milk—for example, I can buy certified, high-grade raw milk in my home state of Washington. If you don't have access to raw, then use the kind of milk (from Twin Brook) I describe in Part 1. Look for non-homogenized vat- or batch-pasteurized whole milk. What you want to avoid is ultra-pasteurized milk or cream, as you will have problems recovering the solids.

This recipe calls for buttermilk. Buttermilk, typically, is the liquid remaining after making butter. Here is a FoodWISE, but sane, moment: making butter itself to yield buttermilk is perhaps too much work for many of us. Buttermilk also can be made by adding a bacteria culture to milk, and heating. Still, I recommend defaulting to "good enough"—buy it in a store (expensive!)—or, make a version of this recipe with just whole milk, and a starter culture you can purchase. For examples and more discussion, see https://wp.wwu.edu/gigiberardi/category/foodwise-resilient-farms-and-nourishing-foods-blog.

Equipment: The simplest equipment is a colander lined with thin muslin cloth, but even a clean handkerchief or thin dish towel will do. You'll need a bowl or pot big enough—at least 2 quarts in capacity—to catch all the whey.

Prep time: Preparation will take a matter of minutes, but fermentation and draining will require several days.

INGREDIENTS

2 quarts buttermilk

PREPARATION

Let milk sit, loosely covered, on the counter at room temperature for 1–2 days until the whey separates from the curds solids.

Pour the mixture into a cloth-lined colander placed over a 2-quart capacity bowl or pot to catch the whey.

Tie up the cloth with a knot so it makes a little sack, which you can then drain, suspended from your kitchen cabinet handle or knob (really, I just use a thick rubber band, tie it around the knot, then hang one end of the rubber band on the cabinet handle—over a bowl it can drip into). Or—if your colander is big and wide enough, and ditto with the receiving bowl—you can just let the mixture drain from the colander into the bowl in which the colander is resting.

Let drain overnight or until the whey is no longer dripping.

Scoop out the soft curds; this is your cream cheese.

Refrigerate the cheese (for up to several weeks) and also the whey (which keeps for some months and can be used for lacto-ferments) in covered Mason jars.

Easy Whey and Yogurt Cream Cheese

Yield: 1 tsp to 1 tbsp whey (depending on how firm the yogurt set is when you buy it), 5 oz cream cheese

You can easily recover whey from commercial whole milk yogurt. This is especially useful when you want just a small amount of whey, for example, for the "Crispy Almonds" recipe below. The yogurt cream cheese is delicious.

Equipment: Muslin cloth or clean handkerchief, medium-sized funnel, and receiving jar

Prep time: Preparation will take a matter of minutes, but fermentation and draining will require a day or two.

INGREDIENTS

8 oz plain whole milk yogurt (organic is a good bet), with no additional emulsifiers or stabilizers or thickeners (which may interfere with your recovery of the solids)

PREPARATION

Line a medium-sized funnel (about four inches in diameter) with a clean cloth or handkerchief and set over a receiving jar.

Add all of the yogurt.

Let drain overnight or until the whey is no longer dripping.

Scoop out the soft curds; this is your yogurt cream cheese.

Refrigerate the cheese (for up to several weeks) and also the whey (which keeps for some months) in covered Mason jars.

GRAINS—WHOLE AND REFINED

Whole grain such as brown rice is a great source of protein, and really is whole. Compared to the list of ingredients on packages of store-bought seasoned rice (hydrolyzed soy protein, brown sugar?), rice simply simmered in a pot looks WISE indeed. If you take the time to inform yourself of what's out there, grains can be very sustainable, too. For example, quinoa seed (not really a grain, but used in dishes as such) has soared in popularity. Just like everything else, when a demand surges, it's hard to meet it, and growers naturally want to jump on the commercial bandwagon in countries like Peru and Bolivia. Issues arise in terms of production methods and land grabs (and clearings) to grow the tasty, high-demand product. But this is when we can rely on certification processes and certified products that come from cooperatives and associations organized to brand their product—and guarantee sustainable production while maintaining availability to local residents at a reasonable cost.

All in all, it's well worth your time to experience grains. Try different combinations and see what your local farmers might have to offer.

Bread

Bread is usually synonymous with the grain it comes from—wheat. Historically, wheat was a mainstay of many family farms: wheat grain would be grown for animal feed and for flour, and the straw used for bedding or construction or returned to the soil. Some grain was saved for seed for the following year, and the crop was used in a rotation that could help break plant disease cycles. Today, commercial wheat seed is much different than it was a hundred years ago—and there are fewer varieties. In the past, literally thousands of varieties of this small grain were available and "grown out" by farmers worldwide, local seeds being the result of adaptation to climate and soils and tastes. Fun fact: It's not difficult to grow your own. Wheat, after all, is a grass. Can you grow grass in your front yard? Yes? Then, chances are you can grow wheat as well. You'd be surprised how much wheat you can grow for flour in a year, in just 200 square feet of good soil. You'd also be surprised how easy it is to mill the grains! You can find small-scale milling equipment for home use available in secondhand markets.

In the United States today, most commercial breads are made with refined flours. Flour is just milled grain. Whole wheat flour is made from the entire wheat kernel. White flour is more processed and more refined to produce a softer, whiter flour. "Bleached" flour is treated with agents like chlorine gas or benzoyl peroxide. Even with "unbleached" white flour, the bran and germ of the kernel have been removed, together with vitamins and minerals (which oftentimes are added back in to "enrich" the flour).

Homemade bread is simple. To the flour, you add yeast and water, and maybe salt and a little sweetener. These are the basics, but commercial store bread has a lot more additions.

Store-bought bread is typically made with industrial-scale white flours (from the wheat "commodity" crops we discussed in Part 1) and commercial yeasts that are used to quickly raise the dough. It is not uncommon for a substance called vital wheat gluten to be added—it helps give bread structure during this extra-fast rising. But according to Stephen Jones of Washington State University's Bread Lab, this ain't bread—and may well be contributing to the digestive discomfort and intolerance we see connected to gluten consumption. Cheap bread, yes, but what is it that we are buying? There's also a hefty dose of chemicals in the bread to act as dough conditioners, emulsifiers, preservatives, and "bread improvers." As for me, I'll take my fermentation slow.

Gigi's Tassajara Bread Redux

Yield: 4 large loaves or 8 small loaves

I found this recipe in 1976, several years after the publication of *The Tassajara Bread Book,* and have been experimenting with it ever since. Because I like to make several dozen small loaves and freeze them, I use large quantities of ingredients. Whole wheat bread freezes fabulously (bread made with white flour may have more moisture in it and can develop frost on the bottom). My little loaves of bread are like a whole meal, with all I fortify them with, and I get them for pennies (compare to the cost of store-bought "natural" breads). When I was busy in graduate school for my dance degree, I would carry three or four little loaves with me for nutritious meals on the go. It was my version of "fast food." However, if you're trying to satisfy picky eaters, you might have to gently introduce them to the heavier whole wheat breads. But honestly, once it comes out of the oven piping hot, with or without butter, no matter what its weight, the bread is hard to resist.

For this recipe, you can add some nuts and fruits and spices to the dough after the second kneading. What I do is roll out the dough again (after I've formed the dough into smaller balls), but not too thin, and add cut apples and dried plums and walnuts and cinnamon and cloves and … whatever sounds good to you. Bring the sides of the dough together and pinch, they'll look like little bowls (of goodness). Voilà! It becomes a favorite potluck food for me! I bake these smaller "sweet loaves" separately as they tend to bake more quickly since the dough is thinner from being rolled out. This bread freezes exceptionally well when protected from dehydration in tightly sealed bags, so I even make double batches of the recipe and then I need to make it less often.

Experiment with gluten-free flours if you like. I haven't done that for this bread, so I'm going to leave those experiments to anyone perusing such cookbooks (there are dozens of recipes for delicious-sounding gluten-free breads). Even if you have some gluten sensitivity, I invite you to consider trying these long-fermentation, whole-grain breads. I myself have a laboratory-certified gluten sensitivity, and my bread doesn't arouse that sensitivity at all. But these days my family enjoys home-baked bread more than I do, as I consume my grains mostly whole and unprocessed. This recipe makes a tremendous amount of bread, as is my wont (see note on this at the beginning of Part 4). Ace bread baker Andrews Inglis has tested this recipe with a smaller amount of flour and grains. It's a delicious version for one 4 × 8-inch loaf and you can find it at https://wp.wwu.edu/gigiberardi/category/foodwise-resilient-farms-and-nourishing-foods-blog.

Equipment: Very large bowl (in a pinch, use a big cooking pot), breadboard for kneading (or clean countertop will do), small mixing bowl, two large baking sheets if you want to make hand-shaped loaves (this is what I do) or bread pans (for four large or eight smaller loaves), parchment paper

Prep time: You're looking at 4 hours from start to finish, including about 3 hours' rising time. Clearly, breadmaking needs to fit into all your other daily activities. It's worth the effort!

INGREDIENTS

½ cup lukewarm water (for the yeast mixture)

1 tbsp yeast (1 pkg) or make your own (a glass jar with flour and water exposed to the air for a few days will capture wild yeasts; for more information, see http://thebreadlab.wsu.edu/going-with-the-grain)

1 tbsp molasses or other sweetener (sweetener is not absolutely necessary, but the yeast mixture rises faster with it. Then again, some people like to add ½ cup or more of the sweet stuff.)

5 cups lukewarm water (with another ½ cup or so water in reserve to add to the sponge)

4 cups unbleached white flour (or a mix of unbleached white or whole wheat; because much of the gluten is in the white flour, using less will give you a slightly denser loaf)

¼ cup extra virgin olive oil (you can substitute butter—about ½ stick, melted, equals ¼ cup) for the mixture, plus more oil for rubbing onto the rising dough and the formed loaves, and for oiling your baking sheets or bread pans

1 tbsp salt

2 cups of any available whole or lightly processed grain you have (I like to use uncooked steel-cut oats, but you can also use wheat berries soaked overnight until soft, cornmeal, or even cooked grains)

6 cups whole wheat flour (and additional flour, as needed)

PREPARATION

First: Making the sponge

The first part of this wondrous process is "making the sponge"—that is, the light, airy dough that ferments with the yeast mixture.

In a small mixing bowl, combine ½ cup lukewarm water with the packaged yeast or a heaping tablespoon of the homemade yeast starter.

Add molasses or other sweetener, stir gently, and set aside.

In a very large bowl, mix 5 cups of the lukewarm water with the 4 cups of unbleached white flour. The mixture should be fairly wet. Don't over-mix.

Add the yeast mixture to the flour mixture, stir just a bit, and let rise in a warm place. Cover bowl with a moist dish towel. If necessary, you can insulate the bowl with a blanket. If it rises too much, you'll have a mess—and not so easy to get out of your towel. It should double in size in about an hour.

Second: Adding all the good stuff to the sponge

I like to "break" the sponge by gently pouring the olive oil and scattering the salt over the beautiful dome of the sponge. Then, fold in the non-flour grains (if adding oats, which are completely dry, you may need to add another ½ cup water to the sponge).

Then fold in whole wheat flour—a cup or two at a time. This dough firms up slowly and you don't want to add too much flour all at once. Stir the sticky dough with a strong wooden spoon. You'll notice the dough is getting drier—go slowly to let the gluten develop. Add flour only to the point where the dough is barely sticky. This can take 10–15 minutes.

Knead the dough. I like to start kneading in the bowl, but then turn it onto a breadboard (be sure to add any scrapings from the bowl) or counter. This dough will be thick! Knead gently, until the dough holds together. There is a possibility the dough will feel too dry; especially if it starts to separate into dough "flakes," then you might need to add some water. If too moist and sticky, you need to add additional flour.

Rub the beautiful dough dome with olive oil and let it rise again for about an hour. You know the drill: leave it covered in a bowl in a warm place to rise.

After one hour of rising (with this much whole wheat flour, the bread will not quite double in size), punch the dough several times (not too much!) and return it to the breadboard or counter for more kneading. Knead gently; the gluten strands are fragile.

Let dough rise for 45 minutes, again in its covered bowl, in a warm place. Note: This last rising gives you a slightly lighter loaf; if you don't want that, skip it and go directly to the steps below.

Third: Shaping and baking

Preheat your oven to 350 degrees, or a little less if your oven "cooks hot." Grease baking sheets or bread pans with olive oil.

Shape mixture into loaves. I like to make 8 smaller loaves—because they are so handy—but you can make 4 large loaves instead. If you use baking sheets rather than bread pans, the loaves do butt up against each other as they bake, which means you have to separate them after cooking (a bit like giant rolls). But I'm not going for looks, I'm going for what works for me. If you want nicely shaped bread loaves, go ahead and use greased bread pans. I admit, they do look prettier.

Rub olive oil lightly over the surface of the loaves and score them (gently slice across the top with a knife, about ½ inch deep—about 3 scores per loaf).

The loaves should rise for another 20 minutes on the sheets or in the pans— but if you find them getting *too* big, use your own judgment as to when they are ready to be put into the oven: That risen loaf is going to be about the same size as the finished loaf.

Bake 30 minutes, then cover loaves with parchment paper to reduce browning.

Bake for another 20 minutes, then test for doneness. Remove one of the sheets/pans and insert a thin knife in a loaf. Does it come out clean? If not, try again after 10 minutes. Of course, each time you remove a loaf from the oven, the temperature lowers and takes a few minutes to go back up.

When the knife comes out clean, remove all the loaves from the oven and let them cool on racks, or any available clean counter space.

You'll be missing out if you don't have a slice of the warm bread just then. The rest? You can freeze loaves in sealed plastic bags (date them!). The loaves will keep for several months, unless someone gets to them first!

NUTS

Nuts are a good source of fats and protein. While you can certainly include them in recipes to produce unexpected combinations, fundamentally there's nothing more Whole than simply eating them as a standalone food. Depending on where you live, local nuts might be available. In the Pacific Northwest where I live, local walnuts and hazelnuts—although not native to this place—abound, making these a very Sustainable option. As always, experiment: Try the "Crispy Almonds" recipe with different nuts.

Crispy Almonds

Yield: 1 lb Crispy Almonds

This is a nice ferment that makes a pound of somewhat sweet, irresistibly textured (in other words, super-crunchy) nuts. This dish, popularized by Nourishing Foods advocate Sally Fallon, also is available in whole food stores as "sprouted" nuts—but you pay for the convenience! You can use whey to kick-start the fermentation. When I use almonds, I most certainly use organic because conventional almonds are miserable for bees. Most almonds are raised on an industrial scale, and pollinated by bees that are raised on an industrial scale as well.

Almonds produced in such proportions depend on the husbandry of a lot of bees, but the bees themselves are managed intensively—often with a variety of treatments to try to control parasites and diseases. At this level of production, it's hard for any natural processes to occur that might help lead to better bee health. It's also hard to produce organic almonds at this scale. As with many foods, finding smaller-scale sources may give you more confidence in the quality of what you're getting and the impacts of producing it.

Equipment: Large bowl for the nuts—with soaking they will double in size! Two baking sheets to spread out the almonds

Prep time: Although the preparation will take only a few minutes, soaking the almonds is an overnight (or all-day) process, as is dehydrating in your oven. This dish can take two days from start to finish—but the flavor and texture reward is extraordinary.

INGREDIENTS

1 lb raw almonds or walnuts (or whatever nuts you can get locally, if that's important to you)

1–2 tsp salt

2 quarts water

Optional: 1 tbsp whey (see recipe for "Easy Whey and Yogurt Cream Cheese," above)

PREPARATION

Add almonds or other nuts, salt, water, and whey (optional) to a large bowl and leave in a warm place overnight. Nuts should swell to about double the size.

Drain and rinse in a colander (you can use the rinse water for cooking soup or stock later). You might need to rinse several times to remove skins.

Set oven on lowest temperature (I use 200 degrees).

Spread almonds evenly over the two baking pans (I don't grease the pans).

Cook until very crisp (for my oven, this usually takes overnight).

Cool completely before storing in a glass container.

Almond Milk

Yield: About 3 cups almond milk

Good colleague and good cook Teresa Rieland of sweetveg.org has created this recipe for FoodWISE.

Equipment: Blender or food processor, fine mesh strainer or nut milk bag (muslin cloth), medium-sized bowl

Prep time: 15–20 minutes (it takes some time to remove peels from the almonds), plus almonds need to soak for 8 hours

INGREDIENTS

1 cup untoasted almonds

3 cups water

PREPARATION

Soak the almonds for about 8 hours or overnight in sufficient water to cover them (they will swell in size).

When done soaking, slip the peels off the almonds and compost (or, spread in garden). Place the peeled nuts in blender or food processor with half the water and blend for a few minutes. Pour this liquid through a fine mesh strainer or nut milk bag and let drain into a medium-sized bowl.

Gather the ground almond pulp out of the strainer or nut milk bag and put back in the blender or food processor with the remaining water. You can repeat this step several times to get more liquid from the pulp and create a smooth milk.

Almond milk keeps for up to a week in the refrigerator.

BEANS

As far as sources of protein go, dried beans are about as Whole as it gets. Beans are food on a most basic level—simply soak dried beans overnight, cook for an hour or two, and you've got a delicious, fibrous protein to which you can add all sorts of toppings, or just eat straight. Beans are also one of the more Sustainable options since, like most legumes, under the right growing conditions they actually benefit the soils they're grown in, rather than strip away nutrients. Dried beans also store easily; they can sit in your pantry for months without going bad. You can have some fun informing yourself about where different varieties come from. Several local farmers at my farmers market offer heritage varieties of dried beans that I've never seen in any store. Go out and experience as many as you can. Your body will thank you for all the delicious protein and fiber.

Vegetarian Chili

Serves 6

I so love a good, hearty chili—and the eggplant here is a worthwhile bonus. Eggplant might seem like an unusual addition, but it adds so much flavor and taste! I enjoy this chili with tender pieces of local beef, but I also love the vegetarian version. I could even imagine a vegan version. Crispy cashews (see "Crispy Almonds" recipe, above) would be a great protein and texture addition, and about a tablespoon of coconut oil would enliven the dish with saturated fat. Use your imagination; the possibilities are limitless! With chili, you can always take a shorter route for preparation: Just open cans of beans and vegetables. The longer route would have you soaking about 1 cup of dried beans (which yields 3 cups of cooked beans) overnight (maybe with a little salt or whey) and cooking them the next day, as well as stewing your own tomatoes (if you have access to ripe ones). Enjoy the simmering step of this recipe, which is definitely worthwhile. In this sweet melee, once you introduce the spices and let them simmer, their bite is just that much softer. The fragrance of the brew indicates that the vegetables are releasing their juices.

Equipment: Large-sized frying pan or cast-iron skillet (at least a 3 quart capacity)

Prep time: Depending on what ingredients you choose to use, this recipe can take anywhere from 75 minutes (the eggplant preparation is a little time-intensive) to a full day if you're soaking dry beans.

INGREDIENTS

1 medium-sized eggplant, unpeeled, cut into ½-inch cubes

¼ tsp salt for drying eggplant

1 tbsp plus 2 tsp extra virgin olive oil, divided

1 large yellow onion (I use the milder yellow onions), chopped

3 cloves garlic, peeled and minced

2 green, red, or yellow peppers cored, seeded, and chopped

1 can (28 oz) Italian plum or any whole tomatoes—or 3 large ripe tomatoes, cored, seeded, and chopped (or, you can use some combination if you really enjoy the fresh tomato flavor)

1–1½ tbsp chili powder

2 tsp ground cumin

4 tsp fresh basil, finely chopped (about 10 leaves) or 2 tsp dried basil

1 tbsp fresh oregano leaves or 1 tsp dried oregano

2 tbsp fresh cilantro, minced

1 tbsp fresh parsley, chopped

Salt and black pepper, to taste

3 cups cooked beans (red kidney, garbanzo, pinto, mixed)—different combinations will change some flavors of the chili

1 tbsp fresh lemon juice

Optional: Add a cup of salsa with the tomato and spices for different flavors.

PREPARATION

Sprinkle eggplant with salt and let stand for 35 minutes; you can use a plate or put directly on a cloth towel; then dry both sides with the towel.

Sauté eggplant in 1 tbsp of olive oil in a large-sized pan or cast-iron skillet over medium heat; when just tender (after about 5 minutes), set the eggplant aside on a plate.

Add 2 tsp more olive oil and heat.

Add onion, garlic, and peppers and sauté until just softened (5–6 minutes).

Add tomatoes, spices, and herbs (and a cup of salsa, if desired); cook uncovered for 20 minutes.

Add the cooked eggplant.

Stir in beans and lemon juice and simmer for another 10–12 minutes.

VEGETABLES

Vegetables provide some of the most FoodWISE options out there. They are Whole from the very start; you don't have to worry about preservatives as long as you're shopping fresh, and even canned veggies are often preservative-free (but high in added salt). Inform yourself about what's available from your neighborhood farms—and while you're at it, do some research on all the amazing nutrients vegetables contain. From vitamin C to iron, vegetables are powerhouses of nutrition. You don't need to memorize which micronutrients are where to make your choices—but you do need to pay attention to Sustainability. Fresh local vegetables can have a low carbon footprint—but many vegetables do require a lot of nitrogen, a limiting factor to production. So scope out integrated farms that recycle nutrients and manage livestock and/or cover crops to ensure fertile soils. Experience—meaning, try—as many different varieties as you can: Experiment with flavors! Chances are, if a recipe calls for something you don't have, you can find something in season to substitute, making all kinds of phenomenal taste discoveries along the way.

Pressure Cooker Vegetable Stew

Yield: About 2¹/₂ quarts stew

Serves 6

When I use my old pressure cooker these days, I'm not just making a meal, I am reliving my early cooking days: from packing up the pot in my parents' home in Los Angeles to bringing it to graduate school in Ithaca, remembering the first times I used it there (admittedly with a little trepidation), then, recalling all the hundreds and hundreds of meals I have cooked in it since. It's what I used almost every day when I was a graduate student. I added my own home-canned tomatoes, my moth-eaten cabbage and broccoli, and all the strong garlic that so easily grew around Ithaca. I fed many people with those meals in my studio apartment: students and neighbors and authors (Frances Moore Lappé, author of *Diet for a Small Planet,* for one), and friends who needed a place to stay (and eat).

I was looking for easy, as these pressure-cooker meals really cooked themselves with just a little veggie washing and cutting (especially the dense carrots or beets). I used butter, then olive oil, and now I am back to butter.

I loved that pressure cooker to death—literally, as I needed to replace the rubber ring that seals the lid several times. I remember, as a twenty-two-year-old student, going into the local Sears for a replacement for the over-stretched ring, and the sixty-something clerk looking at me with wide eyes: How could someone wear out that rubber seal? Easy, just cook with it every day. I wore out ring after ring—that's how much I used it. And getting the right replacement size was sometimes difficult.

So, how does this little miracle of a machine work? Inside the pressure cooker, the boiling point is increased a little, to 230 degrees or so (typically, it's 212 degrees for water at sea level). That higher temperature (still lower than the lowest setting on a Crock-Pot) cooks the food more quickly, with less water loss. Plus, any heat-sensitive nutrients are exposed to high temperatures for that much less time. It's also more efficient in terms of the amount of fuel used. Be aware that, in the cooking, a little perfumed steam is released, not a lot, and the stronger the scent, the closer the stew is to completion. That little rocking pressure valve produces the most friendly sound: Dinner is close.

Thinking FoodWISE, what does that pressure pot do to Whole? Heat-sensitive nutrients, like vitamin C, take a big hit, but they suffer in other types of cooking, too. Nutrients in grains do better, and the fiber count pretty much stays the same. I nevertheless figure that I balance those pressure cooker meals (which are fewer and fewer these days) with a lot of fresh vegetables—sometimes a pound or two a day, for I love salads.

When my pressure cooking was at its peak, I got the vegetables from my friends' organic gardens (or my own), and experimented with vegetables and cooking times, adding grains and spices. Those meals were fast and inexpensive, giving me the time I wanted to focus on my friends and guests—the dining experience itself, rather than the preparation and the cleanup. This was a big bonus to my otherwise busy graduate student and teaching life. The recipe here produces a nice tangle of vegetables. One trick is to cut harder, denser vegetables that take a longer time to cook into smaller pieces.

Note on equipment: If the idea of a pressure cooker is a little daunting for you, you could try this recipe in a Crock-Pot. You can just plug in a Crock-Pot or slow cooker and then not think about it for a few hours. The physical-chemical principles are completely different, but the end product is similar: a one-pot meal. In a Crock-Pot, however, the dish may take about 6 hours to complete.

Equipment: 4-quart pressure cooker

Prep time (for all the chopping and cutting): about 20–25 minutes, plus about 10 minutes for cooking and 10–20 minutes for cooling

INGREDIENTS

¼ cup extra virgin olive oil

4–8 cloves of garlic, peeled and minced

1 large onion, coarsely chopped

1 cup water

1 can (28 oz) whole tomatoes, including draining liquid (or 1 quart-sized jar of home-canned tomatoes)

3 medium carrots, sliced into ½-inch pieces

½ large acorn squash or about 1 pound of other hard-skinned squash, cut into 1-inch pieces

½ medium cabbage, coarsely chopped

½ large bunch kale or chard, coarsely chopped

½ tsp each salt and black pepper, or to taste

PREPARATION

Rinse and prepare the vegetables.

To prepare the squash: cut in half lengthwise; scoop out pulp and seeds; cut one of the halves lengthwise again (into quarters), and then again (into eighths); slice off skin and discard; then cut the squash into 1-inch cubes.

Add olive oil to pressure cooker (ample to coat onions and garlic).

Sauté garlic and onion (uncovered), until onions are somewhat soft and garlic starts to brown.

Add water, then tomatoes, then the rest of the vegetables.

Add salt and pepper and mix.

Seal the lid, and cook on high heat until the pressure gauge starts to wiggle; lower the temperature—you want it to wiggle but there should be little escape of steam.

Cook for 10 minutes after pressure is reached (i.e., the pressure valve is rocking steadily).

Remove from heat and wait 10–20 minutes for the pressure and temperature to lower. I sometimes check for this by ever so slightly tilting the pressure valve. If there is no release of steam, you're ready to remove the lid. You can expedite the cooling process by running cold water over the pressure cooker, but be careful not to dislodge the pressure valve.

If I want to make the stew a little richer with some saturated fat, I add butter and cheese. That's right—to the finished product—it all melts. Coconut oil would also make a good addition.

Baked Garlic

Serves 4

Baked garlic is one of my favorite "entertainment" dishes to make, either at home or for a potluck elsewhere—it is so easy and delicious. It is an excellent way to use a lot of my favorite allium (the family of onions, leeks, and chives). The garlic comes out soft, sweet, and sticky—perfect for spreading on bread or vegetables, or combining with hummus or other spreads, or mixing into a salad dressing. Right now, I am writing in a place where I can get only imported garlic—from China. Indeed, China now provides over 75% of total world production. It's not clear whether that stunning total comes at a hefty price in terms of social costs. Admittedly, the cloves are huge—however, I enjoy most using my own homegrown, simply because it is so tasty.

The sweet taste of the garlic is perfectly complemented with creamed, soft, or hard cheeses, creating a huge medley of taste sensations. I serve the garlic bulbs on a tray, with soft cheeses and coarsely textured grainy breads. Squeezing the baked garlic out of the peels is half the fun—let your guests squeeze and spread the garlic themselves. In this recipe I provide a delicious variation.

Equipment: Fancy terra cotta garlic-baking dishes are available, but all you really need is a glass or ceramic baking dish with lid.

Prep time: 5 minutes, and about 45 minutes for baking

INGREDIENTS

4 large bulbs of garlic, with about ¼ inch cut from the top of the cloves, keeping the cluster of cloves together. There's no need to peel the cloves.

2 tbsp extra virgin olive oil

PREPARATION

Preheat oven to 400 degrees.

Place the prepared garlic bulbs in a glass or ceramic baking dish, cut side up. Drizzle with olive oil and cover.

Bake for about 45 minutes. You can check for tenderness by inserting a knife or fork into a clove.

Remove lid and serve with side dishes—cheeses, breads, and veggies.

GLORIA'S VARIATION

To make the garlic more like a thick spread: After garlic is baked, remove peels, gently press into a paste and add 1 tsp molasses (optional), ⅛ tsp black pepper, and some dried or fresh marjoram and parsley to taste.

Dilly Beans

Yield: 5 quarts

This is one of my staples—my go-to food for potlucks. Friends love these beans. It's really a family recipe (and project), and we have a lot of fun preparing the dilly beans together. I harvest the beans, and my partner and I both prepare them for canning (trimming off the ends, cleaning them). I prepare the garlic and spices, and he the water bath. It is a good division of labor. Note that quantities can be scaled up or down to match how many beans you have. We tend to pack our jars quite loosely and we trim very little from the beans. For a tighter, more uniform pack, you will need fewer jars.

Equipment: You will need a canner or very large pot (with a rack to lower and raise the jars into and out of the water), jar tongs, a large-sized saucepan, a small-sized saucepan, and 5 wide-mouth quart canning jars with metal lids and rings.

Prep time: I won't lie, this can be a half-day affair, depending on how much cleaning your crispy, barely ripe beans require.

INGREDIENTS

10 cups water, plus about 2 cups water to sterilize metal lids and rings

10 cups white vinegar

1½ tbsp salt

1½ tbsp red pepper flakes

5–10 cloves garlic, peeled

5 fresh dill heads or 2 tbsp dill seed

Approximately 3 lbs fresh, crisp yellow wax beans—green and purple beans also work (note that you will be happier with the quality and longevity of the processed beans if you use very crisp, barely ripe beans)

PREPARATION

Clean jars (dishwasher or hand wash).

Fill large canning pot with water and bring to a boil. Use sufficient water to cover your jars when they're sitting on the rack; fill with extra water just to be sure—you can ladle out any extra as you put in the jars, so it doesn't overflow.

Combine water, vinegar, and salt in a large-sized saucepan; bring to a boil (and maintain the boil).

Bring 2 cups water to boil in the small-sized saucepan. Add metal lids and rings, boiling per manufacturers's instructions to sterilize.

Add to each jar: at least ¼ heaping tsp red pepper flakes, 2 cloves garlic (or just 1 if the cloves are large), and 1 head fresh dill and/or 1 generous tsp dill seed.

Pack beans lengthwise/vertically into jars, leaving ¼- to ½- inch head room.

Pour hot vinegar/water/salt mixture over beans, leaving ¼-inch head room.

Hand-tighten lids, then back off rings just a smidge.

Using rack and tongs, immerse jars in boiling water bath and process for 10 minutes.

Lift rack and remove jars carefully with tongs, set apart from each other to cool. If lids don't pop down, put those jars in a refrigerator; the beans start to "pickle" within a few days and will be good for at least a few weeks or more. If jars seal, they can be kept on a cool, dark shelf for months.

Let stand 2 weeks before eating.

Roasted Vegetables

Yield: Quantities are for two large baking sheets (I like to roast a lot at a time)

Serves 2-4

Prepared and cooked well, this recipe gives you wedges of slightly firm beets, potatoes, carrots, and onions. But, if you're not careful in preparing (that is, cutting to the right sizes) and roasting these succulent morsels, you run the danger of ending up with sweet, mushy, charcoal-like vegetable tidbits, rather than the sizeable chunks of delectable vegetables that they should be. You can experiment with the sweetness of the vegetables, adding balsamic vinegar (this will make them quite sweet, depending on the length of roasting time), or merely adding a bit of salt to bring out the flavor (my preference). I also like to experiment with red wine vinegar—not so sweet, and great tang.

FoodWISE, it helps to harvest at the peak of maturity—roots having been fed with nourishing manures and/or composts, maybe even with a celestial connection as in biodynamic practice. Understanding when and why and how our food arrives on our table really matters in the case of vegetables— we tend to eat them whole anyway, much of the flavor being innate: the sweetness of potato and yam, the rustic taste of mature beets (my favorite vegetable), the fruitiness of carrots. The recipe I include here is with one of my favorite combinations of vegetables.

Note on cooking time and temperature: I roast at 375 degrees. This may be a little low, but I like a longer, more controlled roast. If you've cut the veggies just right, both mushrooms and beets can take about the same time, 15–30 minutes.

Equipment: Large-sized mixing bowl, two medium-sized baking sheets (or one very large sheet)

Prep time: About 20–40 minutes, depending on how clean your vegetables are to begin with and roasting time

INGREDIENTS

¼ cup extra virgin olive oil (or you can use more flavorful coconut oil, but roast at a lower temperature)

½ tsp each salt and black pepper per baking sheet, or to taste

2 carrots, sliced into 1-inch pieces

5–10 asparagus spears (not too thick)

2 beets, cut into small wedges

3 all-purpose potatoes (like Yukon gold), cubed

1 onion, cut into wedges

¼ cauliflower, cut into florets

¼ broccoli, cut into large florets (these cook quickly, so you'll want a larger size floret)

10 brussels sprouts, cut in half

10 medium-sized mushrooms

2 green peppers, cored, seeded, and cut into large chunks

Optional: Other root and vine vegetables such as parsnips, turnips, rutabagas, squash—either in thin slices or small wedges

Optional: Herbs that hold up well when baking can be a tasty addition, like fresh rosemary (use a full sprig), fresh thyme (several small sprigs), or 1 tsp each dried rosemary and thyme per sheet

Optional: 2 tbsp fresh parsley, chopped

PREPARATION

Preheat oven to 375 degrees.

Put ¼ cup olive oil and salt and pepper in a large bowl. Add vegetables and toss until they are lightly coated.

Transfer vegetables to the two baking sheets (or, one very large sheet) and sprinkle with herbs, if desired. Make sure there is a little space around each piece.

Set the sheets on the middle or lowest racks in the oven. Check at 15 minutes by removing sheets from the oven and stirring the vegetables (turning over individual pieces, if possible). Return to oven.

Check every 7–8 minutes. Use a knife or fork to check for doneness.

Transfer to glass serving dishes, and immediately stir in chopped parsley if you like. Note that these tasty vegetable morsels can be served either hot or at room temperature.

Avocado Guacamole

Yield: 2-3 cups

Serves 6

For years in Los Angeles, I took avocados for granted; I lived with a huge avocado tree in the backyard, and had a dancer's big appetite to go with it. Avocado featured prominently in just about everything I cooked: egg frittata with gobs of avocado and cream cheese (the industrial-scale kind—before I made my own), toast (from my whole-grain Tassajara loaves) with smashed avocado and seeds of various kinds, chicken with avocado smear, smoothies with avocado—and, of course, guacamole. Guacamole, for me, is FoodWISE—a poster food for Wholeness: the avocados themselves, with coarse salt and pepper, hefty amounts of cumin and other spices, raw garlic and onion (made practically invisible by mincing and dicing, or fully exposed in large wedges so you know precisely what you are eating), ripe tomatoes (not overly ripe, you certainly don't want the guac to be runny, right?). My whole family enjoys guacamole;

my son and I love it with hefty amounts of onion and lots of tomatoes, but that much onion is not for everyone. Sometimes I add a spicy salsa. Delicious.

Equipment: Small mixing bowl

Prep time: About 15 minutes

INGREDIENTS

2 large ripe avocados

2 cloves garlic, peeled and minced (or cut into larger pieces, if you like)

¼ onion of your choice, minced (or cut into larger pieces, if you like)

1 large ripe tomato, cut into small wedges (if ripe tomatoes are out of season, you can substitute a few tablespoons of tomato-based salsa)

1 tsp cumin, or to taste

2 tbsp fresh cilantro, finely chopped

½ lime, juiced

½ tsp each salt and black pepper, or to taste

Optional: 2 tbsp spicy salsa

PREPARATION

Cut avocados in half, remove the seed, scoop out the fruit into a small mixing bowl.

Add remaining ingredients (and spicy salsa, if desired). Mix well, but not so the mixture is runny. Enjoy with fresh vegetables, or breads.

BROCCOLI GUACAMOLE VARIATION
Yield: About 2 cups

Emphasizing different ingredients changes the taste profile. You would think the avocado itself would be essential—for the creamy fat it provides. But substituting some cooked vegetables, like broccoli, creates a reasonable facsimile. The salt+-pepper+other spices+vegetable is a substantive, irresistible combination. Know that this is a dish where if you skimp on the salt, you will be sorry. Mashing and stirring: You want to be a little gentle in how you add and stir, to avoid an unappealing mush. This recipe won't have quite the smooth feel of the usual avocado version, but it is definitely tasty. There's a bonus: If you mix all in a blender or food processor, you have a delicious salad dressing.

Equipment: Vegetable steamer basket in a medium- or large-sized cooking pot with a lid, small mixing bowl

Prep time: 30–40 minutes, depending on cooking time for broccoli

INGREDIENTS

1 medium head broccoli, cut into florets (this will cook to about 3 cups)

1–2 tsp water

Other ingredients same as for "Avocado Guacamole," without the avocado

Optional: Splash of red wine (or other) vinegar or spoonful of salsa

PREPARATION

Steam the broccoli using the steamer basket in approximately ½–¾ cup of water. Cover the pot when steaming. When broccoli is tender, remove from heat. This should take just a few minutes.

While the broccoli is cooling, prepare the other ingredients.

When cooled, gently mash the broccoli with a fork into a small mixing bowl with 1–2 teaspoons of water.

Add remaining ingredients, as given in the "Avocado Guacamole" recipe, including the wine vinegar and/or salsa if desired.

Vegetarian Curry

Serves 6 (depending on whether you have rice, yogurt, and/or other side dishes)

Here is your chance to experiment with new spices. Experiment, too, with their sautéing time. Or experiment with heating them without oil, to draw out more of the flavor. And try using different vegetables; I often make this curry with whatever is in the fridge that needs to be cooked. That said, I must admit that I am particularly fond of nightshade-family flavors like eggplant, potato, green pepper, and tomato. Add these vegetables toward the end of cooking, and you'll get a delicious matrix, aided and abetted by carrots, onions, and cauliflower. The taste symphony is quite extraordinary. You could use mostly canned or frozen veggies, but in-season fresh veggies provide some serious flavor and texture. This can be served with grain (rice, millet) and some processed fruit (chutney or fruit relish), although the recipe's raisins or plums should provide a sufficiently sweet flavor. A simple raita—a yogurt with finely cut vegetables—complements the spiciness of the dish.

Equipment: Large-sized pan or skillet, small mixing bowl

Prep time: About 65–75 minutes (there's a lot of vegetable cutting and fussing; if using dried chickpeas, add soaking time to prep time)

INGREDIENTS

1 lb eggplant (approx. 1 large eggplant), cut into 1-inch cubes

Salt (enough to sprinkle generously on raw eggplant cubes)

1 tbsp plus 2 tsp extra virgin olive oil, divided—you also can use coconut oil

2 large cloves garlic, peeled and minced

1 large onion, thinly sliced

2 medium carrots, thinly sliced

2 large potatoes, diced

1–2 green peppers, thinly sliced

½ large head cauliflower, cut into bite-sized florets

4–5 firm, ripe medium-sized tomatoes, chopped (save any liquid) (if you don't have fresh ripe tomatoes, consider using a 28-oz can of whole tomatoes)

½ cup vegetable stock (see "Vegetable Stock" recipe, below)

1 can (16 oz) chickpeas (garbanzos), drained (or use 1 cup dried chickpeas, soaked overnight, then simmered for about half an hour)

¼ cup raisins (or ½ cup chopped dried plums)

Optional: plain yogurt for garnish

Spices

1 tsp curry powder (mild, hot, or both), or to taste

1 tsp ground cumin

1 tsp ground ginger

½ tsp turmeric

¼ tsp cayenne pepper

¼ tsp ground cinnamon

¼ tsp ground coriander

1 tsp each salt and black pepper, or to taste

PREPARATION

Mix spices in small mixing bowl and set aside.

Sprinkle eggplant with salt and let stand for 35 minutes; you can use a plate or put directly on a cloth towel; then dry both sides with the towel.

While the eggplant is sitting, prepare the other vegetables.

Then heat 1 tbsp olive oil over medium heat in a large skillet. Add the eggplant and cook, stirring often, for about 5 minutes. Remove eggplant from the pan, set aside leaving the oil in the pan.

Add the spices and garlic to the pan and sauté for several minutes.

Add 2 tsp more oil to the skillet, then add onion, carrot, potatoes, green pepper, and cauliflower.

Lightly sauté the vegetables for 5–8 minutes—they should be *al dente* (firm).

Add tomatoes, including liquid, then add stock.

When vegetables are heated through, add chickpeas and raisins or dried plums, then the cooked eggplant; heat thoroughly.

Serve with yogurt (optional).

Fried Cauliflower

Serves 4

Another one of my favorite ways to use eggs is for this lightly fried cauliflower. It actually is more of a sauté—quickly cooked in a small amount of olive oil. I think this is delectable; it's my mother's recipe, and a huge hit at my numerous potlucks. (As I remember, my mother fried the cauliflower more than I would want to.) Its prominent ingredients (and smells) are of steamed cauliflower and cumin—and plenty of cumin, at that. I cook the cauliflower (divided into florets) until barely soft (that's a big part of the deliciousness of the dish—the *al dente*–textured cauliflower). Then I roll it all in a gummy mixture of eggs and milk, a little whole wheat flour or ground corn, doused with salt, pepper, and a lot of cumin; and heat gently.

Equipment: Vegetable steamer basket in a medium- or large-sized cooking pot with a lid, two medium mixing bowls, large-sized frying pan or cast-iron skillet

Prep time: About 30–35 minutes, depending on the cooling time for the cauliflower

INGREDIENTS

1 medium head cauliflower, broken or cut apart into large florets

2 large eggs

¼ cup milk

1 cup whole wheat flour or coarse cornmeal

1 tsp garlic powder (I like to use garlic powder as it blends well with the flour or cornmeal)

2 tsp cumin, or to taste

½ tsp each salt and black pepper, or to taste

PREPARATION

Steam the cauliflower using the steamer basket in approximately ½–¾ cup of water. Cover the pot when steaming. Do not overcook—florets should be firm. Cool to room temperature.

Mix eggs and milk in medium-sized bowl.

Combine whole wheat flour or coarse cornmeal and spices in separate medium-sized bowl.

Dip (I use my hands) cauliflower pieces in egg-milk liquid. Slosh them around until covered.

Then roll cauliflower pieces in dry ingredients.

Sauté on medium heat until heated through or just slightly browned.

Nice food extender: Toward the end of cooking, you can add the remaining egg mixture to the frying pan—it's all yummy—as well as more salt, pepper, and cumin. Note that this dish is delicious served hot, or at room temperature.

Italian Greens

Serves 4

The first time I tasted these strong greens, I was in Umbria, Italy's "green heart." The cook was Ann Martini, who had been enculturated into Italian cooking with the help of the Italian family she married into. This simple recipe couldn't be easier: steam the greens, squeeze out the excess water (this is key), sauté some diced garlic, then add the tender greens with plenty of salt and pepper. The greens have a little bite to them—pungent, too, from the olive oil and the earthy garlic.

Note on serving: This dish is also good at room temperature.

Equipment: Vegetable steamer basket in a medium- or large-sized cooking pot with a lid, large-sized frying pan or cast-iron skillet

Prep time: About 12–15 minutes

INGREDIENTS

1 bunch of hearty greens (chard, kale, mustard, turnip, and/or collard greens), washed and chopped

2 cloves garlic, peeled and minced

½ tbsp extra virgin olive oil

¼ tsp each salt and black pepper, or to taste

Optional: ¼ lemon

PREPARATION

Using the steamer basket in approximately ½–¾ cup of water, steam greens until tender, about 5 minutes. Cover the pot when steaming.

Squeeze out all the water (preferably, over a bowl—you can capture liquid from the greens this way and save it for stock).

In a large-sized frying pan or cast-iron skillet, heat oil and sauté the minced garlic for about a minute.

Add greens and cook until heated through, about 2–3 minutes. Use a fork to separate the greens.

Add salt and pepper.

Serve with a squeeze of lemon (optional).

Vegan Salads and More

I lived in a small town in Switzerland as I was finishing this book—and the *padrone* of my boarding house was a gourmet vegan. The diversion that those long lunches gave me was invaluable. At least a half hour to prepare, and definitely a half hour (or more) to clean up, but the food was delicious and enjoyable. Those amazing lunches followed a formula of sorts:

SALADS

These consisted of: sliced lettuces and various greens, carrots, onion, fresh herbs that I'd just picked on the grounds of the beautiful Goetheanum where I worked, all in a coconut-yogurt-horseradish dressing or a raw green smoothie dressing. And, oh yes, don't forget to add some micro-greens (i.e., sprouts of various sorts).

VEGETABLES/VEGETABLE COMBINATIONS

Discover cauliflower! A most memorable dish for me was a barely steamed giant cauliflower head—intact! We then finished this "cauliflower roast" in the oven—covered first with almond milk. The almond milk gave the cauliflower a gentle crust—so different from the typical dairy (cheese and butter) dousing for cauliflower. The sweet cauliflower taste was memorable—try it for yourself!

Also experiment with these vegetable combinations:

Sliced beets, carrots, and onions—lightly cooked in a little bit of water—with no oil.

Chickpeas—soaked overnight, then simmered for 10 minutes with diced potato.

Polenta heated in a skillet with a little tahini (a paste made from sesame seeds) and vegetable stock.

Green peppers (just lightly steamed) stuffed with hummus (cooked garbanzo beans blended with tahini, garlic, and lemon juice).

Lentils cooked in diced tomatoes.

Squash cooked in freshly made tomato juice.

GRAINS

On occasion, we added grains: rice cooked for 15–20 minutes in coconut milk and heated for another 5 minutes in the oven.

SOMETHING SWEET

Every now and then, we enjoyed a wonderful concoction of fresh lemon and orange (from Spain or somewhere else in the European Union; always barely peeled, so there would be quite a lot of "white" remaining—adding pungency to the concoction), with slices of apple, pear, and persimmon with *flohsamenschalen* (psyllium husks). These ingredients would be pureed and refrigerated, and topped with a beautiful ground cherry and coconut yogurt.

Whole Roasted Cauliflower

Serves 6-8

Thanks to Teresa Rieland of sweetveg.org for creating this recipe for FoodWISE, based on my first-person account of those long lunches in Switzerland.

Equipment: Vegetable steamer basket in a medium- or large-sized cooking pot with a lid, baking sheet or large-sized cast-iron skillet, small cup, parchment paper

Prep time: 25–30 minutes

INGREDIENTS

1 head cauliflower, whole and washed

¾ cup unsweetened almond milk (see "Almond Milk" recipe, above)

½ tsp salt

PREPARATION

Remove any leaves and cut the stem flush with the bottom of the cauliflower so it will lie flat on the baking sheet.

Using the steamer basket in approximately ½–¾ cup of water, steam the cauliflower until just barely tender, taking care not to overcook it—about 10–12 minutes (turning over, midway through) depending on the size of the cauliflower. Cover the pot while steaming. Test for doneness by piercing the cauliflower with a knife—there should be slight resistance.

Place a rack in the top third of the oven and turn the oven on to broil.

Stir together the almond milk and salt in a small cup.

Place cauliflower stem side down on a parchment-lined baking sheet or in a cast-iron skillet. If your cauliflower won't stand up, it can be rested on its side. Using a spoon, coat the cauliflower with about ¼ cup of milk mixture. Place in oven to broil.

Broil for a few minutes, then remove partially or fully from the oven to pour ¼ cup more of the milk over the cauliflower, making sure the cauliflower is coated. Return to the oven and let broil a few minutes more, watching carefully to ensure that it does not burn.

Add the remaining almond milk. Continue to broil until the top of the cauliflower is golden brown. Remove from oven and serve as one beautiful, giant head.

STOCKS AND SOUPS

A good stock is an excellent foundation for soups and sauces, adding substantial flavor. Soups complement that whole-food bread you are now making in giant quantities. They're the alchemic result of leftover vegetables and meats (and fruits! You'll be a believer if you try a medley of summer fruits in an orange base—and topped with some cultured milk product).

Stocks are easy to make. Meat stocks consist of basically parboiling chicken remains or fish scraps or beef bones, and teasing the nutrients out with a little bit of vinegar or other acid, until you have a rich broth. For vegetable stocks, just simmer vegetables! Check the garden to harvest some ripe vegetables, and think about that low carbon footprint!

The possibilities for variety in soup are endless. Begin with oil or animal fat or a small amount of water in a large pot (look at Goodwill, the Salvation Army, or other secondhand shops to purchase large pots), and sauté or otherwise heat any number of vegetables—try leeks and onions, then add celery, and later zucchini (cut), cabbage (finely torn), cauliflower (florets), and/or mushrooms (leave whole, or cut in half). Add some water, and gently simmer until vegetables are barely soft. Keep track of what vegetables you use in making the soups; you're going to learn a lot. And most important, of course: enjoy!

Chicken Stock (with Boned Meat)

Yield: 2-3 quarts

This is my mother's simple recipe for chicken stock: straightforward and practical. It also yields a lot of boned meat—useful for chicken salad, enchiladas, spicy shredded chicken, and taco fillings. These days we use our own chickens. We aim for heritage breeds, although in the past we have raised Cornish Cross. And yes, our chickens run around freely, and eat organic grain.

Equipment: Large-sized saucepan (4–6 quarts) or 6-quart stockpot with cover, slotted spoon, fine mesh strainer or colander

Prep time: 2.5–3 hours

INGREDIENTS

1 pastured chicken (about 3½–4 lbs in weight)

1–2 tbsp butter

2–3 quarts water

2 onions, quartered

2 carrots, in 1-inch slices

2 green peppers, cored, seeded, and quartered

Mixed herbs (thyme, marjoram, oregano, rosemary, sage), either several fresh sprigs or ½ tsp dried each

PREPARATION

Clean chicken and cut into large pieces.

Heat butter in saucepan or pot until almost melted.

Sauté chicken until lightly brown, turning frequently.

Add water to cover and simmer. I like to have the lid partially ajar when simmering.

Once water is simmering, add onions, carrots, green peppers, and mixed herbs. (After cooking the chicken, this liquid becomes the rich stock.)

After 20–25 minutes of simmering, check to see that the chicken is cooked. The meat should pull away easily from the bone.

If the chicken is cooked, and leaving vegetables to simmer, remove chicken and cool so it can be easily boned.

Pull meat from the bones, and store it in the fridge until ready for use.

Add bones back to the stock and simmer, partially covered, for an additional 2 hours or more to recapture more nutrients. During simmering, use a spoon to skim off any foam that rises to the surface.

Remove bones, vegetables, and herb stems with a slotted spoon, then strain the remaining liquid through a fine mesh strainer or colander.

From my mother: "Leave stock in fridge overnight. Use it as the liquid in which to cook rice, or by itself to soothe you when you are sick." Right.

Actually, the stock can last several days in the fridge and at least 4–6 months when frozen in sealed bags or glass jars (just be sure to leave a generous amount of headspace).

Vegetable Stock

Yield: 2-3 quarts

The range of vegetables you can choose for vegetable stock is indeed great— good, delicate flavors won't be overpowered by the sweetness of animal fat, as in a meat stock. Gather as many fresh or leftover vegetables as you can (avoiding those that might render odd tastes, like artichoke leaves).

Equipment: Large-sized saucepan (3–4 quarts) or 6-quart stockpot with cover, slotted spoon, fine mesh strainer or colander

Prep time: 2–3 hours

INGREDIENTS

1 tbsp extra virgin olive oil

1 onion, quartered

2 carrots, cut into 1-inch slices

2 stalks celery, cut into ½-inch slices

1 leek (all parts, except roots), thinly sliced

2–3 quarts water

2 tbsp vinegar (red wine or white)

2 tomatoes, in wedges

1 cup mushrooms, whole

½ cauliflower, coarsely chopped

Mixed herbs (marjoram, oregano, rosemary, sage, thyme), either several fresh sprigs or ½ tsp dried each

2 handfuls of fresh parsley, coarsely chopped, or 2 tbsp dried

2 bay leaves

½ tsp each salt and black pepper

PREPARATION

The stock can be made with or without first sautéing the vegetables (if you're not sautéing, you don't need oil); experiment with the flavors that result from each method.

Heat olive oil in saucepan or pot over medium heat.

Add onions, carrots, celery, and leek. Sauté for several minutes. Stir occasionally.

Add water and vinegar, bring to a boil, then lower temperature to a simmer.

Add the remaining vegetables, herbs, parsley, and bay leaves. Cover and simmer for several hours.

Using a fine mesh strainer or colander, strain the stock.

Compost the "spent" vegetables that remain.

The stock can last several days in the fridge and at least 4–6 months when frozen in sealed bags.

Lentil and Mint Soup

Serves 6-8

This recipe comes from one of our student potlucks (thank you, Sarafina!).

This recipe calls for medium-sized leeks. If you cannot find leeks, you can substitute green onions, white onions, or shallots. Note that with leeks, the dark, green leaves are going to be a little tougher than the white and light green part of the leaves; I use them all (and compost the root). To wash, separate the layers of leaves under water.

Equipment: Large mixing bowl, colander, large-sized saucepan with cover

Prep time: About 40–50 minutes; lentils need to soak 6–8 hours

INGREDIENTS

2 cups dry lentils

6 cups water for soaking lentils

8 cups plus 2 cups vegetable (or chicken) stock (see Stock recipes above), divided

1 tbsp red wine vinegar

2 tsp coriander seeds, crushed

3 medium-sized leeks, thinly sliced

1 tbsp fresh cilantro, chopped

2 tbsp fresh mint, coarsely chopped

¼ tsp each salt and black pepper, or to taste

PREPARATION

Sift through the lentils to remove any small bits of rock or dirt. (It is much easier to pick out stones right at the beginning, before lentils are wet.) Rinse well and soak in the 6 cups of water in a large bowl for 6–8 hours or overnight. Soaking is not absolutely necessary for lentils, but it will reduce the cooking time. Strain in a colander and recycle the soaking liquid (use on indoor or outdoor plants).

Cook lentils in the 8 cups of stock, first bringing to a gentle boil, then simmering for about 20 minutes, during which time you can add red wine vinegar and coriander. Add more water or stock as needed while the lentils are cooking. You may need to add as much as 2 cups of extra liquid to cook the lentils completely.

When the lentils are starting to get soft, add the leeks, cilantro, mint, salt, and pepper. Continue to simmer until the lentils are fully cooked. You may want to add additional salt or red wine vinegar, to taste.

Serve and enjoy!

Butternut Squash Soup

Serves 4-6

This hearty soup is delicious any time of the year. Note that the zest is from the outer part of a citrus peel (for this recipe, be careful not to grate the skins too closely to the white part, which is bitter). Serving roasted squash seeds atop the soup makes it even more delicious. This soup is easily reheated.

Equipment: Baking sheet, parchment paper, blender or food processor, large-sized saucepan, zester (you can also use a vegetable peeler or knife)

Prep time: 1.5 hours

INGREDIENTS

2 medium butternut squashes, halved and seeded

4 cups vegetable (or chicken) stock (see Stock recipes above)

1 medium lemon, juiced (about 2 tbsp)

1 cup milk (or use heavy cream for a thicker soup)

2 tsp grated orange zest

1 tsp ground coriander

½ tsp each salt and black pepper, or to taste

4 tsp fresh cilantro, chopped

PREPARATION

Preheat oven to 400 degrees.

Cut squash in half, scoop out the seeds (save these to roast in the oven on a parchment-lined baking sheet—at about 400 degrees for about 20–25 minutes—sometime after you have cleaned away the pulp), and place squash halves face-down on a baking sheet lined with parchment paper. Bake until soft, about 45–55 minutes.

Let the squash cool, then scrape the squash meat off the skin with a large spoon.

Put half the squash meat in a blender or food processor with half of the stock and half of the lemon juice and puree it. Move puree to saucepan. Repeat with the other half of the squash, stock, and lemon juice.

Reheat on stove until heated through, then remove from heat.

Stir in the milk or cream, orange zest, coriander, salt, and pepper.

Before serving, add the cilantro for garnish.

MEAT

Meat—is it FoodWISE? Meat is a Whole food when you get it fresh from the woods or the farm. Some of the recipes below could use meat you can hunt yourself: it's hard to get a smaller carbon footprint than with wild-harvested venison, especially if you don't travel far to get it. Farming your own meat is also an option—or, if it's not an option for you, try finding a local farmer who raises meat in a Sustainable way. Visit the place your chickens were raised. Do you feel okay about the lives of the animals there? If so, you can WISEly support humane meat production. If not, find a smaller farm—or set up a chicken coop of your own.

Roasted Chicken
Serves 4

My very favorite way to roast chicken is adapted from a *New York Times* recipe. I've hosted many a chicken taste test, and this recipe usually wins. We roast our own chickens, and the rich smells permeate the house, especially when I open the oven door to baste the skin. The chicken sizzles and I know that the basting juices are doing their job of creating a golden crusty coating. We add our dried plums and figs, inside the cavity or even outside in the pan; they are irresistible!

Equipment: Roasting pan or large baking pan (I use a large glass baking dish), kitchen twine, turkey baster or large spoon

Prep time: 10 minutes, plus refrigerator time and 50–60 minutes for roasting

INGREDIENTS

1 pastured chicken (about 3½–4 lbs in weight)

2–3 tbsp each salt and black pepper, or to taste

Mixed herbs, in the form of leafy sprigs—we take whatever is in our garden: tarragon, thyme, marjoram, oregano, and plenty of rosemary and sage (these are to stuff the cavity of the bird, so you'll need some hefty sprigs, or use ½–1 tsp each of different herbs)

PREPARATION

Preheat oven to 425 degrees.

Season the chicken inside and out with the salt and pepper (I use plenty of both and rub them on with my fingers).

Leave the chicken in the refrigerator overnight, if you can manage that; however, even an hour or two will help in developing some of the flavor. In a pinch, just stick it in the oven (after placing herbs in the open cavity, see below).

Place chicken breast-side up in a roasting pan. Next, place all the herbs in the open cavity and tie the legs together with kitchen twine to avoid drying out the slower-cooking parts of the chicken (this is ideal; but it will be good enough if you simply leave the legs as they are).

Roast for 45–50 minutes, basting the chicken periodically with the pan juices using a turkey baster or large spoon. When done (about another 10 minutes), the juices should run clear (not pink) when the thigh is pierced with a knife. Let sit for 5–10 minutes before serving.

Butterflied Leg of Lamb

Serves 6

This recipe is from my longtime friend and dance buddy, Judy, in Trumansburg, New York. The marinade with the acid, the rosemary, and the Dijon mustard is a winning combination—try it!

A word or more on the lamb you use. If you Google "feedlot lamb," mostly you get ads or university/government notices about the details of finishing lambs (by feeding them grain) in feedlots. But sheep didn't evolve to eat a grain-based diet with little to no fresh grass; or have a prolonged, final feeding with grains. Look around for yourself—talk to your local butcher, seek out a farmers market, or make friends with somebody who has pastured sheep. Become Informed, and you can make this meal Sustainable and Whole.

Lots of Whole ingredients go into this meal, from—ideally—the lamb itself to the spices to the olive oil. As for Experience, this dish provides a great opportunity to interact with the farmers in your agricultural web. Plus, it's an experience well worth tasting. Lamb meat tastes like little else, in part due to its fat content. But it takes some experience to learn to cook it properly. This recipe takes away some of the guesswork—the marinade is phenomenal (mustard, soy sauce, ginger, garlic, red wine vinegar) and the meat tenderizes in it, so little broiling is necessary.

Note: You want the lamb butterflied (either by a butcher or you can do it); the meat is cut in half lengthwise and laid flat for quicker cooking. If you have a bone-in leg, either cut the meat off the bone carefully, or cut it off one side of the bone, and spread it out before marinating.

Equipment: Large-sized bowl, and large roasting or large glass baking dish

Prep time: 15 minutes, plus marinating time and 30 minutes for cooking

INGREDIENTS

¼ cup extra virgin olive oil

⅓–½ cup Dijon or other coarse mustard

2 tbsp soy sauce

1 tbsp fresh or dried rosemary (you can add more for a more fragrant dish, including adding fresh sprigs on top)

2 tsp fresh ginger, grated (if you only have ground ginger, substitute with ¼ tsp)

4 cloves garlic, peeled and chopped

A few generous dashes of red wine vinegar (other vinegars will do) or juice from ½ lemon

1 leg of lamb (most likely, you will find one about 4 lbs, more if bone-in; see note above)

Optional: additional 4–8 cloves garlic

PREPARATION

Mix together in a large-sized bowl the olive oil, mustard, soy sauce, rosemary, ginger, garlic, and red wine vinegar or lemon juice.

Prepare the lamb by rinsing and drying.

Optional: You can add 4–8 cloves additional garlic by cutting ½-inch slits in the meat and inserting cloves. If the cloves are relatively large, you may need to slice some of them before inserting.

In the bowl, add lamb to mixture and marinate for several hours or overnight. Turn lamb at least once while marinating.

Remove lamb from marinade and scrape off remaining marinade (some people like to leave the marinade on, but the mustard will char in the oven).

Place lamb in a large roasting pan or large glass baking dish (my preference).

Place an oven rack in the upper middle position and preheat broiler for 7–10 minutes.

Broil lamb until done, about 12–15 minutes per side (for rare / medium rare).

FISH

With everything I've written about factory farming and fisheries, you might think I'd caution against eating fish. Here in the Pacific Northwest, we do enjoy a relative abundance of some species of marine fish—some so fresh we can eat it as sushi. As we discussed in Part 1, sustainable fishing is a big issue for both saltwater and freshwater species. Farmed fish actually often aren't the best solution—sustainable wild-caught salmon is a good addition to a FoodWISE menu.

Marinated Salmon

Serves 4

You'll notice that each of the five species of Pacific salmon goes by at least two common names. A typical whole fillet might be about 1–1½ pounds, or more if the species of salmon is larger. A king/chinook is larger than a coho/silver, which typically is bigger than a red/sockeye salmon—and their fillets will be correspondingly different in size. If the fish are harvested and handled well, the less fatty (and less expensive) fish like chum/keta and pinks/humpies are a good Whole, Informed, Sustainable—and affordable—choice.

I like to use marinades for fish, but depending on how fresh and flavorful the fish is, you may want to omit them. Here's a favorite marinated salmon recipe, cooked *en papillote* (in paper) to effectively steam the fish.

Equipment: A large mixing bowl, one large-sized baking dish, parchment paper

Prep time: 1 hour

INGREDIENTS

2 medium lemons, juiced (about 4 tbsp)

¼ cup extra virgin olive oil

2 tbsp balsamic vinegar

¼ cup melted butter

¼ tsp cayenne pepper

2 tbsp dill weed

2 8-oz salmon fillets, rinsed (with skin)

Salt and black pepper, to taste

Additional herbs, for cooking: fresh rosemary and sage sprigs (or ½ tsp each, dried)

PREPARATION

Mix all ingredients (lemon juice, olive oil, vinegar, melted butter, cayenne pepper, and dill weed) except additional herbs in a large mixing bowl.

Add fillets and marinate for 30 minutes, turning at least once.

Preheat oven to 375 degrees.

Remove fillets from marinade and place skin side down onto parchment paper in a clean baking dish.

Sprinkle fish with salt, pepper, rosemary, and sage.

Bring up the sides of the parchment paper; I wrap the fish by simply folding it over the fish and tucking under any loose ends.

Bake on the lowest rack of the oven for about 20 minutes. Fish is done when the meat flakes.

Potato and Shrimp Salad with Peas

Serves 4-6

Moist, juicy peas are so easily grown in the garden—but, let these vines go unattended and the seeds will eventually solidify into pure starch. Of course, this might be your intention: the seeds dry easily in their pods on the vine and maybe you want to save them to plant next year. This recipe calls for a cup of the juicy seeds—whether fresh, canned, or frozen. Of course, steaming, canning, pressure sealing, and then bouncing along a bumpy interstate can seem like an industrial-style assault, but you can use canned peas for a casserole and the dish is still tasty. The peas do a little better with flash freezing: they endure a blast of frigid air, bob along in ice water, and then spill into packages and bags. They're still peas, and still good food.

Fresh pea substitute: If you can't find fresh peas, consider using fresh sugar snap peas—usually easy to find in stores. Concerned about the source of those out-of-season veggies? Try to find some closer to home.

Either processed or fresh, "cooked until tender" means just that—don't overcook. To test for doneness, take a fork with thin tines, and puncture one of the peas on the top of the pile in your saucepan.

Equipment: Vegetable steamer basket in a medium- or large-sized cooking pot with lid, large-sized saucepan, large mixing bowl

Prep time: 20–25 minutes, plus 10–15 minutes for shelling peas if you are using fresh, and 20 minutes for peeling and deveining shrimp

INGREDIENTS

8 small red potatoes, cut into medium-sized cubes (I do not remove peels—but wash thoroughly, depending on source, if not removing)

1 lb fresh shrimp

1 cup shelled fresh green peas

2 tsp extra virgin olive oil

1 jalapeño pepper, stemmed, seeded, and minced

¼ tsp each salt and black pepper, or to taste

PREPARATION

Using the steamer basket in approximately ½–¾ cup of water, steam the potatoes for about 20 minutes or until cooked. Set aside.

Steam peas for about 2–4 minutes or until just tender. Set aside.

Steam shrimp for about 3 minutes. Let cool, then peel away shells, and "devein" (pull or cut away) the thin dark strip from the back of the shrimp (obviously, you can use frozen, or even canned, shrimp and skip this step entirely—just be informed as to where that convenience food is coming from).

Combine all ingredients in a mixing bowl or directly into a serving dish. Serve hot or cold.

SWEET

Sweet is a tough topic. We've already looked at Robert Lustig's work on fructose, especially in terms of sweeteners added to processed foods. For some, sugar is a terrible trigger (as is alcohol)—an invitation to overeat and overdrink. It doesn't help that in the United States we elevate after-dinner sweets to full-course status. Friends, this is not the same in other parts of the world, where anything sweet after a meal is a delicacy—and served in very small amounts. There's something else, too. Less sweet can translate into more flavor, as with this recipe for Pear Almond Pudding.

Pear Almond Pudding

Serves 4

This recipe is from Teresa Rieland of sweetveg.org.

Equipment: Blender or food processor, medium-sized pot with lid, small mixing bowl, baking sheet

Prep time: 15–20 minutes; almonds need to soak for 8 hours

INGREDIENTS

½ cup untoasted almonds, divided into two ¼-cup portions

3 medium-sized pears

2 tbsp water

⅛ scant tsp salt

PREPARATION

In a small mixing bowl, soak ¼ cup almonds in water, covered, overnight or at least 8 hours. Remove and compost the skins.

Core the pears and chop them into chunks. Leave the skins on.

Place pears in a medium-sized pot with 2 tbsp of water. Add the soaked almonds and salt.

Bring to a low simmer, cover, and cook until the pears are soft.

Lightly toast the other ¼ cup of almonds (spread on a parchment-lined baking sheet and roast for about 3–4 minutes at 350 degrees), then chop coarsely. These will be used for a topping.

When the pears are done cooking, place in a blender or food processor and puree until smooth and creamy.

Spoon into serving dishes and top with the toasted almonds.

Salted Chocolate Hazelnut Bark

Yield: About 30 pieces

This is from one of our larger potlucks. Thank you, Mona!

Fall is the time of year for hazelnuts in the Pacific Northwest. Hazelnuts are tasty and local, yet I admit I can break my locavore principles for a good piece of chocolate. I enjoy the crunch of this chocolate combination, and the nutty texture of the finished bark.

Getting away from sweet: In some recipes for chocolate-nut bark, the nuts are first candied (by adding sugar to the melting butter); I forgo that step here, and advise that if you really want to get away from sweet, use chocolate that's 85% or 90% cocoa solids (with little added sugar). This will give you bark with a zing!

Equipment: Rolling pin, baking sheet, parchment paper, double boiler (just a saucepan fitting into or atop another saucepan of boiling water)

Prep time: This can take 45 minutes or longer. Plan on about 20 minutes for roasting the nuts.

INGREDIENTS

1½ cups raw hazelnuts, shelled (about 3 cups in the shell)

1 tbsp unsalted butter

1 lb dark chocolate, finely chopped

1 tsp salt (for sprinkling)

PREPARATION

Roasting the nuts

Preheat the oven to 350 degrees.

If necessary, shell the hazelnuts. Compost the shells.

Roast the nuts in a single layer on a parchment-lined baking sheet for about 10 minutes (very fresh nuts may take longer), until they are lightly golden. Ensure there is air space around each nut.

Wait a few minutes to cool, then wrap the nuts in a kitchen towel for a minute. Rub vigorously in the towel to remove the majority of the skins, which you can then compost.

Let cool to room temperature, then crush hazelnuts somewhat with a rolling pin. Set aside.

Preparing the nuts

Warm butter in a saucepan on stove until melted.

Add roasted hazelnuts; stir until well coated.

Transfer to the same parchment-lined baking sheet, spreading out to separate nuts.

Let cool. Break up any clumps of nuts.

Set aside ¼ of the nuts.

Preparing the chocolate and bark

Break the chocolate into small pieces.

Heat chocolate in double boiler until melted, 7–10 minutes.

Remove from heat, add nuts from baking sheet directly into the double boiler, and stir quickly to combine.

While still hot, spread chocolate-nut mixture on same baking sheet (this baking sheet and parchment paper are getting a lot of use), keeping nuts in a single layer.

Top with the ¼ cup of the nuts you set aside.

Sprinkle with salt.

Chill until chocolate is set, about 3 hours.

Break bark into pieces and store between layers of parchment or waxed paper. The bark will keep in the refrigerator for about a week.

VARIATIONS

Feel free to add flavor or spices to the melting chocolate: vanilla extract or powder, or cinnamon or peppermint oil.

Dandelion Wine

Yield: About 4 quarts

Sugar and alcohol are triggers for some people and, if that's you, then this recipe could deliver a double whammy: caution advised.

I've been making dandelion wine (inspired by Ray Bradbury's famed novel) for thirty-five years, ever since I first got a recipe from my dear friend Loretta. With this wine, more than anything else, I've taken the time to observe differences in all that I do when making a particular batch. The date on the bottle reminds me of the warm day when I first gathered the dandelion flowers. Uncorking it, as in Bradbury's book, is intoxicating, with the smallest sounds and feel of that spring or summer day flooding my memory. I still have wine from decades ago, and I have wine made in the year my children were born—1996.

In preparing the wine, I have made my fair share of mistakes! Time has been on my side, though, to help correct them, figure out what I did right, and duplicate and build on the beautiful formula as best I can. A few edits of note: The batches that are slightly bitter, from earlier in the season, are a tonic extraordinaire. So, reduce the sugar, and its bitterness will scream "tonic" to you. Or experiment with how much of the dandelion plant you use; the more green stem you include, the more bitter.

Serve the brew at its rightful temperature: *really cold*. I so look forward to that first sip, pursing my lips ready for the cold trickle—almost always in the company of good friends—and usually in tiny amounts as an after-dinner "digestive."

The Wholeness is from the dandelions (wild harvested of course), lemon and orange (or try lemon balm, a mildly citrus-scented herb). Use cane sugar. You can even make your own yeast by letting a mixture of flour and water ferment on your kitchen counter for a few days (see "Gigi's Tassajara Bread Redux").

This wine becomes somewhat alcoholic soon after it starts to ferment. Be sure to keep the covered stone or glass crock in a clean and dry place (a kitchen counter works well) so as to avoid unwanted bacteria or yeast.

If you can refrain from adding much additional sugar, you will have a stimulating beverage with quite a bite. Otherwise, you'll get a small shock at how much sugar the fermentation can devour. I rarely consume sweet, but if I do, it's here.

Equipment: Large-sized pot, fine mesh strainer or colander, large stone or glass crock for fermenting, muslin cloth or clean handkerchief, medium-sized funnel, and bottles with corks or lids

Prep time: Approximately 30 minutes to harvest dandelions and 50 minutes for preparation; 2 weeks to ferment; an hour or two to strain solids and bottle.

INGREDIENTS

1 quart dandelion blossoms, stems removed (picked after the petals are open and the morning dew has dried)

4 quarts water

1 pkg dried yeast (or ferment your own moist microbial slurry)

½ cup warm water

1 lb seedless raisins (or any other dried fruit; I've tried 1 lb plums, which are local for me)

6 cups (3 lbs) cane sugar

1 lemon and 1 orange, unpeeled, cut into small pieces (if substituting lemon balm, add a huge bunch of it, thoroughly rinsed)

PREPARATION

Pick clean, fresh dandelion blossoms.

Place blossoms in 4 quarts water. Bring to a boil, then simmer vigorously for 30 minutes.

Cool a bit, then strain through a colander into large stone or glass crock to remove blossoms. Let liquid stand until cool.

Dissolve yeast in ½ cup of warm water. Wait 5 minutes.

Add yeast mixture (if you're using a home microbial ferment, add about a tablespoon of it to the mixture), raisins or other dried fruit, sugar, lemon, and orange (or lemon balm) to the dandelion liquid.

Let stand for 2 weeks, covered but not tightly; stir every day (an unparalleled sweet, alcoholic aroma will greet you!).

Strain through muslin cloth or handkerchief several times until clear.

Pour into bottles; put corks in loosely (in case it continues to ferment).

Date bottles and store on a cool, dark shelf—you'll want to remember and refer to the day you bottled up this spring delight.

NOTES

INTRODUCTION

Page 1 **and distribute it**

"Food web" is commonly used in ecology as a metaphor for the prey–predator relationships found in a particular ecosystem. Those relationships make up food chains, which taken together form a network. The term is decades old and is important in describing ecological communities in terms of energy flows. But the agricultural web, encompassing the production of human food and livestock feed, and all that we require to grow, process, and distribute it, is a little different. Here, we aren't talking about a natural chain of predators and prey.

Page 2 **United States Department of Agriculture (USDA) dietary guidelines**

See the following example from Caroline L. Hunt, "Food for Young Children" pamphlet, United States Department of Agriculture Farmers' Bulletin 717, (March 4, 1916): 1–2, "Food for children between three and six years of age should be chosen with reference to their bodily needs. [This would include] at least one food from each of the following groups: milk and dishes made chiefly of milk.... Meat, fish, poultry, eggs, and meat substitutes. Bread and other cereal foods ... butter and other wholesome fats, vegetables and fruits, simple sweets." See also: Caroline L. Hunt and Helen W. Atwater, "How to Select Foods I. What the Body Needs" pamphlet, United States Department of Agriculture Farmers' Bulletin 808, (March 1917): 7, "But unless small amounts of specially fat materials, like butter, oil, or cream, are used, the meals are likely to be lacking in it." Finally, see USDA Center for Nutrition Policy and Promotion, "A Brief History of USDA Food Guides," June 2011.

Page 5 **Carlo Petrini writing about "Slow Food"**

Carlo Petrini, trans. Clara Furlan and Jonathan Hunt, *Slow Food Nation: Why Our Food Should Be Good, Clean, and Fair* (New York: Rizzoli International Publications, 2013).

Page 5 **Finding Balance**
Gigi M. Berardi, *Finding Balance: Fitness, Training, and Health for a Lifetime in Dance,* 2nd edition (New York: Routledge, 2005). The first edition, with shorter title, appeared in 1991.

Page 5 **and Be Wary**
Eat, Drink, and Be Wary (Churchill Films, 1979), educational film strip audio, 15 min, www.youtube.com/watch?v=UhF2_T7pLSk.

Page 9 **and consumed."**
Julie Guthman, *Weighing In: Obesity, Food Justice, and the Limits of Capitalism* (Berkeley, CA: University of California Press, 2011), 19.

Page 9 **The End of Food**
Paul Roberts, *The End of Food* (Boston: Houghton Mifflin Company, 2008).

Page 9 **The "Whole" farm**
I use the word "whole" a lot in this book. Usually, it is not capitalized (as in "whole food"). This is also the case for the other words that form the WISE acronym, "informed," "sustainable," "experience" (or, "experience-based thinking," which I use interchangeably). Rather, I capitalize such words when they appear in the same sentence (or close to it) as "Food-WISE"—or when I am talking about their larger meaning in the FoodWISE approach to making food choices, as here—The "Whole" farm.

Page 9 **should not be washed**
Does washing the raw chicken increase your chances of getting food poisoning from campylobacter bacteria? See National Health Service, "Why You Should Never Wash Raw Chicken," www.nhs.uk, June 17, 2017. Also see U.S. Food & Drug Administration, "Food Safety Tips for Healthy Holidays," November 27, 2017.

Page 10 **in the case of rice**
Rice production and trade have additional hidden costs in the form of barriers to trade for poorer countries due to US rice subsidy policies artificially bumping up the price. See Daniel Griswold, "Grain Drain: The Hidden Cost of U.S. Rice Subsidies," Trade Briefing Paper 25 (Cato Institute Center for Trade Policy Studies, November 16, 2006).

Page 10 **arsenic in rice**
Questions about arsenic in rice provide interesting study. Rice has a tendency to take up arsenic, but also there might be a "poison legacy" from persistent arsenic-based chemicals used on previously sown cotton fields. See also Mark Peplow, "US Rice May Carry an Arsenic Burden: Legacy of Cotton Pesticides Might Be Poisoning Crops," *Nature,* August 2, 2005, https://doi.org/10.1038/news050801-5.

Page 10 **seasonal, and sustainable**
The acronym for fresh, local, organic, seasonal, and sustainable is FLOSS, coined by Henning Sehmsdorf of S & S Homestead on Lopez Island. See http://sshomestead.org/farm.

Page 11 **us non-gardeners**
Techniques for making a garden in a sack are described in numerous websites, for example: www.instructables.com/id/A-garden-in-a-sack.

Page 12 **Should we care?**
See Tina Bellon, "U.S. Judge Tosses Lawsuits about Labels on Parmesan Cheese," Reuters, August 24, 2017.

Page 14 *Tassajara Bread Book*
Edward Espe Brown, *The Tassajara Bread Book* (Boston: Shambhala, 1970).

Page 15 *What America Eats*
Steve Ettlinger, *Twinkie, Deconstructed: My Journey to Discover How the Ingredients Found in Processed Foods Are Grown, Mined (Yes, Mined), and Manipulated into What America Eats* (New York: Hudson Street Press, 2007).

Page 18 **number of confined animals**
For one definition of a CAFO, see United States Environmental Protection Agency (US EPA), "Regulatory Definitions of Large CAFOs, Medium CAFO, and Small CAFOs."

Page 18 **integrity farming."**
Integrity farming is discussed widely in Joel Salatin's many books, but also found on his website, Polyface: The Farm of Many Faces, 2018, www.polyfacefarms.com.

Page 19 **any different**
Physiologically, biochemically (in terms of the actual animal); this actually is a smaller concern for me compared to questions about glyphosate and also socioeconomic impacts of the technology.

Page 19 **kill harmful bacteria**
See, for example, the general discussion in Chris Erchull and Laura Fisher, "Remedying and Regulating the Unintended Consequences of Subtherapeutic Dosing of Livestock with Antibiotics: Can the EPA's Implementation of the Clean Water Act Rein in the Problem," *Western New England Law Review* 38, no. 3 (2016): 397–423. Similar concerns worldwide are in Chetan Sharma, Namita Rokana, Mudit Chandra, Brij Pal Singh, Rohini Devidas Gulhane, Jatinder Paul Singh Gill, Pallab Ray, Anil Kumar Puniya, and Harsh Panwar, "Antimicrobial Resistance: Its Surveillance, Impact, and Alternative Management Strategies in Dairy Animals," *Frontiers in Veterinary Science* 4 (January 8, 2018), https://doi.org/10.3389/fvets.2017.00237.

Page 19 **aided by Marjorie Spock)**
See a thoroughly interesting narrative on this developed by Dan McKanan, and drawing on the work of others. Dan McKanan, *Eco-Alchemy: Anthroposophy and the History and Future of Environmentalism* (Oakland, CA: University of California Press, 2018).

Page 19 "Dirty Dozen"
Environmental Working Group, "EWG's 2019 Shopper's Guide to Pesticides in Produce," March 20, 2019.

Page 20 turn-of-the-century millhouse
H. W. Quaintance, "The Influence of Farm Machinery on Production and Labor," *Publications of the American Economic Association* 5, no. 4 (1904): 1–106.

Page 22 of ourselves."
M. F. K. Fisher, *How to Cook a Wolf* (New York: World Publishing, 1942).

PART 1

Page 27 into the biodynamic movement
Rudolf Steiner Archive & e.Lib, "About Rudolf Steiner," www.rsarchive.org.

Page 27 the nation's soil resources
Douglas Helms, "Conserving the Plains: The Soil Conservation Service in the Great Plains," *Agricultural History* 64, no. 2 (Spring 1990): 58.

Page 27 interest in sustainable farming
Masanobu Fukuoka, *The One-Straw Revolution: An Introduction to Natural Farming* (Emmaus, PA: Rodale, 1978).

Page 28 produces carbon emissions
"Sources of Greenhouse Gas Emissions," Overviews and Factsheets, US EPA, December 29, 2015.

Page 28 increased to five million acres
"State Fact Sheets: United States," USDA Economic Research Service (ERS), March 6, 2019.

Page 28 1% of all arable (farmable) land
"United States—Arable land (% of land area)," Trading Economics, https://trading-economics.com.

Page 28 "some" of what they eat is organic
Kristen Bialik and Kristi Walker, "Organic Farming Is on the Rise in the U.S.," *Pew Research Center,* January 10, 2019.

Page 29 and conserve biodiversity."
"Organic Production and Handling Standards Fact Sheet," USDA, November 2016.

Page 29 such as California Certified Organic Farmers
"CCOF: Organic Certification, Education and Outreach, Advocacy and Leadership since 1973," California Certified Organic Farmers (CCOF), www.ccof.org.

Page 29 up to 5% may not be)
"Organic Production," USDA, November 2016.

Page 30 **protecting organic farmers**

See information on this topic: Betsy Greene, Casey Giguere, Rebecca Bott, Krishona Martinson, and Ann Swinker, "Case Study of Contaminated Compost: Collaborations between Vermont Extension and the Agency of Agriculture to Mitigate Damage Due to Persistent Herbicide Residues," Livestock and Poultry Environmental Learning Community.

Page 32 **family-scale farming community,"**

"Cornucopia Institute—Economic Justice for Family Scale Farming," Cornucopia Institute, www.cornucopia.org.

Page 32 **environmental impact is contested**

Mike Berners-Lee, *How Bad Are Bananas?: The Carbon Footprint of Everything* (Vancouver: Greystone Books, 2011).

Page 34 **form of agricultural use**

"USDA ERS—Ag and Food Statistics: Charting the Essentials. Land and Natural Resources," USDA, October 26, 2018.

Page 34 **its own definitions**

See Robert Hoppe, "U.S. Farms, Large and Small," USDA, January 13, 2015.

Page 35 **in terms of farm debt burdens—economic sustainability**

Devanik Saha, "Farm Debt Crisis: 70% of Agricultural Families Spend More than They Earn," *Business Standard News,* June 27, 2017.

Page 35 **production by larger farms**

Robert Hoppe, "Structure and Finances of U.S. Farms: Family Farm Report, 2014 Edition," USDA ERS, December 2014.

Page 36 **11% of US agricultural output**

J. M. MacDonald and R. A. Hoppe, "Large Family Farms Continue to Dominate U.S. Agricultural Production," USDA ERS, Statistic: Farm Economy, March 6, 2017.

Page 36 **3% of sales**

"Farm Economics: Value of Production, Number of Farms, and Income down Slightly," 2017 Census of Agriculture Highlights, ACH17-1/April 2019, USDA National Agricultural Statistics Service.

Page 37 **federal tax incentives**

Gigi M. Berardi, Rebekah Paci-Green, and Bryant Hammond, "Stability, Sustainability, and Catastrophe: Applying Resilience Thinking to U.S. Agriculture," *Human Ecology Review* 18, no. 2 (2011): 115–25.

Page 37 **suffer declining profit margins**

Rebekah Paci-Green and Gigi Berardi, "Do Global Food Systems Have an Achilles Heel? The Potential for Regional Food Systems to Support Resilience in Regional Disasters," *Journal of Environmental Studies and Sciences* 5, no. 4 (December 2015): 685–98, https://doi.org/10.1007/s13412-015-0342-9.

Page 37 important case study
Gigi M. Berardi and Charles C. Geisler, eds., *The Social Consequences and Challenges of New Agricultural Technologies,* Rural Studies Series (Boulder: Westview Press, 1984); with credit to the important early work of Andrew Schmitz and David Seckler, O. E. Thompson, and Ann F. Scheuring in California; and Leon B. Perkinson and Dale M. Hoover in the southeast United States.

Page 39 began in 1845
The "Great Famine" led to the death of about one million Irish from starvation and disease and the emigration of one to two million more. And, in fact, heavy reliance on one variety of potato—the Irish Lumper—may have contributed to the severity of the famine, because of the Lumper's susceptibility to the previously unknown strain of blight disease *Phytophthora infestans.* However, the other varieties of potatoes grown at the time besides the Lumper also were susceptible. The real problems were almost total dependence by a large, poor population on potatoes (that dependence itself had economic, social, and political causes), and the virulence of the potato blight. See Cormac Ó Gráda, "The Lumper Potato and the Famine," *History Ireland* 1, no. 1 (Spring 1993); Barbara Maranzani, "After 168 Years, Potato Famine Mystery Solved," History.com, October 19, 2018. After nearly two centuries, scientists have identified the plant pathogen that devastated Ireland, killing one million people and triggering a mass emigration.

Page 39 risk losing entire species
Shanna Carpenter, "Q&A with Cary Fowler: Saving Seeds to Protect Our Food Supplies," *TED Blog,* September 2, 2009.

Page 40 billion in sales
Barbara Farfan, "The World's Largest Supermarket Chains 2018," The Balance Small Business, December 16, 2018.

Page 40 sales in 2017
National Retail Federation, "STORES Top Retailers 2018," *STORES: NRF's Magazine,* https://stores.org/stores-top-retailers-2018.

Page 40 influence on local employment
Michael J. Hicks, "Job Turnover and Wages in the Retail Sector: The Influence of Wal-Mart," *Journal of Private Enterprise* 22, no. 2 (Spring 2007): 137–60.

Page 41 aspects of chicken production
Annie Lowrey, "What Does Monopsony Mean? Chicken Farms Offer an Answer," *The Atlantic,* September 4, 2018.

Page 41 enter Chicken McNuggets
See a journalistic critique in Mark Bittman, "Is Junk Food Really Cheaper?" *New York Times,* September 24, 2011.

Page 41 world of fast food in 1983
Roberts, *End of Food,* 46.

Page 41 largest seller of chicken
Forty-six million pounds a year, supplied by Cargill, according to one source: "How Many Chickens Are Killed Each Year to Accommodate McDonald's Products?" McDonald's Canada, Our Food, Your Questions, June 23, 2012. By the way, if you still want chicken nuggets, it's actually not difficult to make your own. And recipes abound. For example: Melissa D'Arabian, "Homemade Chicken Nuggets," Food Network, www.foodnetwork .com. For the main ingredient, you should be able to find humanely and organically raised chicken in stores.

Page 42 "Shared Values and Guiding Principles"
"UM Dining," accessed May 8, 2019, www.umt.edu/dining/default.php.

Page 42 one of the most thorough critiques
Paul Roberts, *The End of Oil: On the Edge of a Perilous New World* (New York: Houghton Mifflin, 2004); Roberts, *End of Food.*

Page 42 along with Harriet Friedmann
Harriet Friedmann, "The Political Economy of Food: A Global Crisis," *New Left Review* 197 (1993): 29–57.

Page 42 Marion Nestle
Marion Nestle, *Food Politics: How the Food Industry Influences Nutrition and Health,* Revised and Expanded Tenth Anniversary Edition (Berkeley and Los Angeles: University of California Press, 2013).

Page 42 Michael Pollan
Michael Pollan, *In Defense of Food: An Eater's Manifesto* (New York: Penguin Books, 2008).

Page 42 and Eric Schlosser
Eric Schlosser, *Fast Food Nation: The Dark Side of the All-American Meal* (New York: Houghton Mifflin, 2001).

Page 42 deconstructed Twinkies
Ettlinger, *Twinkie, Deconstructed;* Gary Taubes, numerous works including *The Case Against Sugar* (New York: Alfred A. Knopf, 2016).

Page 42 impressive investigative reporting
For example, Maryn McKenna, *Big Chicken: The Incredible Story of How Antibiotics Created Modern Agriculture and Changed the Way the World Eats* (Washington, DC: National Geographic, 2017).

Page 42 to academic articles
For example, Michael Carolan, *The Real Cost of Cheap Food,* 1st edition, Routledge Studies in Food, Society and the Environment (New York: Earthscan, 2011); or Jennifer

Clapp and Caitlin Scott, "The Global Environmental Politics of Food," *Global Environmental Politics* 18, no. 2 (April 4, 2018): 1–11, https://doi.org/10.1162/glep_a_00464.

Page 42 **to nonprofit advocacy**
For example, see "Resource Library," Center for Science in the Public Interest.

Page 42 **Academic Julie Guthman**
Guthman, *Weighing In.*

Page 43 **that are feeding the world's livestock**
Simon Fairlie, *Meat: A Benign Extravagance* (White River Junction, VT: Chelsea Green Publishing, 2010).

Page 43 **even citrus, fruit, almond, and cotton industries**
Fairlie, *Meat,* 27.

Page 44 **animals become infected**
Jon Henley, "Welfare Doesn't Come into It," *The Guardian,* January 5, 2009; Earl B. Shaw, "Swine Industry of Denmark," *Economic Geography* 14, no. 1 (1938): 23–37, https://doi.org/10.2307/141556; Tina Struve, "Risk Assessment of Antimicrobial Usage in Danish Pig Production on the Human Exposure to Antimicrobial Resistant Bacteria from Pork" (Technical University of Denmark, 2011).

Page 44 **restrictions on such use**
M. Ganzler, "Europe's Move on Antibiotic Use in Livestock Leaves U.S. in the Dust Again," *Forbes,* November 1, 2018.

Page 44 **work on the subject**
Michael C. Appleby, V. Cussen, L. Garces, L. Lambert, and J. Turner, eds., *Long Distance Transport and Welfare of Farm Animals,* 1st edition (Wallingford, UK: CABI, 2008).

Page 44 **written about large confinement chicken**
"Chickens," United Poultry Concerns: Promoting the Compassionate and Respectful Treatment of Domestic Fowl; "Food Consumption and Nutrient Intakes," USDA ERS, October 20, 2016; Felicity Lawrence, "If Consumers Knew How Farmed Chickens Were Raised, They Might Never Eat Their Meat Again," *The Guardian,* April 24, 2016; A. A. Olkowski, "Pathophysiology of Heart Failure in Broiler Chickens: Structural, Biochemical, and Molecular Characteristics," *Poultry Science* 86, no. 5 (May 2007): 999–1005, https://doi.org/10.1093/ps/86.5.999; Yiqun Wang, Catherine Lehane, Kebreab Ghebremeskel, and Michael A. Crawford, "Modern Organic and Broiler Chickens Sold for Human Consumption Provide More Energy from Fat than Protein," *Public Health Nutrition* 13, no. 3 (March 2010): 400–408, https://doi.org/10.1017/S1368980009991157; Kathy Shea Mormino, "Prolapse Vent in Chickens: Causes & Treatment," The Chicken Chick; Morgan Brennan, "Inside Sunrise Farms' Avian Flu Chicken Slaughter," CNBC,

April 24, 2015; "Animal Manure Management: RCA Issue Brief #7," Natural Resources Conservation Service, December 1995.

Page 44 **a new record**
K. Jones, M. Haley, and A. Melton, "Per Capita Red Meat and Poultry Disappearance: Insights into Its Steady Growth," USDA ERS, June 4, 2018.

Page 44 **and we want it cheap**
Keri Szejda Fehrenbach, Allison C. Righter, and Raychel E. Santo, "A Critical Examination of the Available Data Sources for Estimating Meat and Protein Consumption in the USA," *Public Health Nutrition* 19, no. 8 (June 2016): 1358–67, https://doi .org/10.1017/S1368980015003055.

Page 45 **problem for our food supply**
For a review of terminology about GE organisms, see P. Byrne, "Genetically Modified (GM) Crops: Techniques and Applications - 0.710," Colorado State University Extension, August 2014.

Page 45 **Roundup Ready corn and soybeans**
For information on products such as soybeans, see "Products|Soybeans|Roundup Ready PLUS," www.roundupreadyplus.com/products/soybeans.

Page 45 **produced and marketed glyphosate**
See Warren Bell, "The Last Roundup: How Monsanto Created the Fable of 'the World's Safest Herbicide,'" *National Observer,* July 25, 2016; Monsanto, "Backgrounder: History of Monsanto's Glyphosate Herbicides," June 2005; "A Short History of Glyphosate," Sustainable Pulse, September 6, 2017. Controversies around glyphosate abound—ranging from notices in the Federal Register (US EPA, "Glyphosate Proposed Interim Registration Review Decision," Federal Register 84, no. 87 (May 6, 2019): 19782–83) to news reporting on controversial rulings against Monsanto/Bayer (Sam Levin and Patrick Greenfield, "Monsanto Ordered to Pay $289m as Jury Rules Weedkiller Caused Man's Cancer," *The Guardian,* August 11, 2018).

Page 46 **raising the risk of some cancers**
Although studies have shown a low hazard potential for glyphosate to, say, mammals, questions remain. See: Luoping Zhang, Iemaan Rana, Rachel M. Shaffer, Emanuela Taioli, and Lianne Shepard, "Exposure to Glyphosate-Based Herbicides and Risk for Non-Hodgkin Lymphoma: A Meta-Analysis and Supporting Evidence," *Mutation Research/Reviews in Mutation Research,* February 2019, https://doi.org/10.1016/j .mrrev.2019.02.001. Review articles suggest that use of varying datasets over differing periods of times could explain some of the diverse views on the safety of the chemical, including its carcinogenic potential for humans. See: Jose V. Tarazona, Daniele Court-Marques, Manuela Tiramani, Hermine Reich, Rudolf Pfeil, Frederique Istace, and Federica Crivellente, "Glyphosate Toxicity and Carcinogenicity: A

Review of the Scientific Basis of the European Union Assessment and Its Differences with IARC," *Archives of Toxicology* 91, no. 8 (2017): 2723–43, https://doi.org/10.1007/s00204-017-1962-5.

Page 46 **already economically vulnerable**
Fred Kirschenmann, G. W. Stevenson, Frederick Buttel, Thomas A. Lyson and Mike Duffy, "Why Worry about the Agriculture of the Middle? A White Paper for the Agriculture of the Middle Project," (agofthemiddle.org, 2008), https://doi.org/10.7551/mitpress/9780262122993.003.0001.

Page 46 **windblown GE pollen alighted on their fields**
Berkeley Tech. L. J, "Monsanto Canada Inc. v. Schmeiser," *Berkeley Technology Law Journal* 20 (2005): 179, https://doi.org/10.15779/Z38WQ2S. Concerns, of course, extend to consumers, too: Michele Simon, "ConAgra Sued Over GMO '100% Natural' Cooking Oils," Food Safety News, August 24, 2011.

Page 47 **referred to as FVH commodities**
Philip Martin and Douglas Jackson-Smith, "An Overview of Farm Labor in the United States" (Western Rural Development Center, Utah State University, 2013).

Page 47 **followed by Florida, Texas, and Washington**
Philip Martin, "Reducing Migration Costs and Maximizing Human Development," in *Global Perspectives on Migration and Development,* ed. Irena Omelaniuk, Global Migration Issues (Dordrecht: Springer Netherlands, 2012), 27-52, https://doi.org/10.1007/978-94-007-4110-2; Philip Martin, "High-Skilled Migrants: S&E Workers in the United States," *American Behavioral Scientist* 56, no. 8 (August 1, 2012): 1058–79, https://doi.org/10.1177/0002764212441786. For an important article on Florida labor relations, see Noam Scheiber, "Why Wendy's Is Facing Campus Protests (It's about the Tomatoes)," *New York Times,* March 7, 2019. Also see Laura-Anne Minkoff-Zern, "Farmworker-Led Food Movements Then and Now: United Farm Workers, The Coalition of Immokalee Workers, and the Potential for Farm Labor Justice," in *New Food Activism: Opposition, Cooperation, and Collective Action,* Alison Alkon and Julie Guthman, eds. (Berkeley, CA: University of California Press, 2017), 157–178.

Page 47 **(excluding California) are 83% foreign-born**
Philip Martin and Douglas Jackson-Smith, "Immigration and Farm Labor in the U.S.," National Agricultural & Rural Development Policy Center, May 2013.

Page 47 **operations relying on it remain vulnerable**
Dennis U. Fisher and Ronald D. Knutson, "Uniqueness of Agricultural Labor Markets," *American Journal of Agricultural Economics* 95, no. 2 (January 1, 2013): 463–69, https://doi.org/10.1093/ajae/aas088.

Page 48 **we won't have farms**
Pam Lewison, "Despite Shortages, Farm Labor Is under Attack Again," Washington Policy Center, January 21, 2019.

Page 48 **make it into the United States at all**
Martin notes in his 2016 article in *AgBioForum* that in 2009, legalized special agricultural workers represented less than 10% of farm workers (down from a high of 40% in 1989), while unauthorized farm workers have hovered around 45%–55% from 1997 to 2009. See Philip Martin, "Immigration and Farm Labor: Challenges and Opportunities," *AgBioForum* 18, no. 3 (2016): 252–58.

Page 49 **Breezy Hill and Stone Ridge orchards**
M. B. Ryan, "Farm Employees Make Decent Wage," personal interview, Stone Ridge NY, September 2018.

Page 51 **within our own country**
Kim Severson, "From Apples to Popcorn, Climate Change Is Altering the Foods America Grows," *New York Times*, May 1, 2019.

Page 51 **biggest source of carbon dioxide in the United States**
"Sources of Greenhouse Gas Emissions," Overviews and Factsheets, Greenhouse Gas Emissions, US EPA.

Page 51 **commodities contribute to this**
"Sources of Greenhouse Gas Emissions," US EPA.

Page 51 **manure produced in livestock operations**
A dairy herd may produce twenty-seven million tons of manure a year (Roberts, *End of Food*, 7). One hog can produce three gallons of feces and urine every twenty-four hours, so one concentrated hog operation can emit as much sewage as a midsize city. See Michael Van Amburgh and Karl Czymmek, "Series: Phosphorus and the Environment, 2. Setting the Record Straight: Comparing Bodily Waste between Dairy Cows and People," *What's Cropping Up? Articles from the Bi-Monthly Cornell Field Crops Newsletter* (blog), June 21, 2017. Ruminant livestock—cows, goats, buffalo, the sheep that I am so fond of—also belch methane as a by-product of their digestion.

Page 51 **soybeans, cattle, sugarcane, and palm oil**
Yale School of Forestry & Environmental Studies, "Sugar Cane, Palm Oil, and Biofuels in the Amazon," Global Forest Atlas, https://globalforestatlas.yale.edu.

Page 51 **Climate Impacts Group (CIG) at the University of Washington**
University of Washington Climate Impacts Group, "Our Work," Climate Impacts Group, https://cig.uw.edu.

Page 51 **intersection of knowledge generation and application."**
University of Washington Climate Impacts Group, "CIG at UW," Climate Impacts Group.

Page 51 **disadvantaged from climate change impacts**
University of Washington Climate Impacts Group, "An Unfair Share: Exploring the Disproportionate Risks from Climate Change Facing Washington State Communities," Climate Impacts Group.

Page 51 *State of Knowledge: Climate Change in Puget Sound*
G. S. Mauger, J. H. Casola, H. A. Morgan, R. L. Strauch, B. Jones, B. Curry, T. M. Busch Isaksen, L. Whitely Binder, M. B. Krosby, and A. K. Snover, *State of Knowledge: Climate Change in Puget Sound* (Seattle: University of Washington Climate Impacts Group, November 2015), https://doi.org/10.7915/CIG93777D.

Page 52 **In our work, but also elsewhere**
Hermine Mitter, Martin Schönhart, Manuela Larcher, and Erwin Schmid, "The Stimuli-Actions-Effects-Responses (SAER)-Framework for Exploring Perceived Relationships between Private and Public Climate Change Adaptation in Agriculture," *Journal of Environmental Management* 209 (March 2018): 286–300, https://doi.org/10.1016/j.jenvman.2017.12.063.

Page 52 **(what happens if current trends continue?)**
Rachel James, Richard Washington, Carl-Friedrich Schleussner, Joeri Rogelj, and Declan Conway, "Characterizing Half-a-Degree Difference: A Review of Methods for Identifying Regional Climate Responses to Global Warming Targets," *Wiley Interdisciplinary Reviews: Climate Change* 8, no. 2 (2017): e457, https://doi.org/10.1002/wcc.457.

Page 52 **farmers are getting worried**
The University of Washington's CIG in February 2019 issued a report summarizing the October 2018 *Special Report on Global Warming of 1.5 °C* by the influential Intergovernmental Panel on Climate Change (IPCC), along with related consequences for Washington State. See A. K. Snover, C. L. Raymond, H. A. Roop, and H. Morgan, *No Time to Waste: The IPCC Special Report on Global Warming of 1.5 °C and Implications for Washington State* (Seattle: University of Washington Climate Impact Group, 2019).

Page 53 *How Bad Are Bananas?: The Carbon Footprint of Everything*
Berners-Lee, *How Bad Are Bananas?*

Page 53 **carbon impacts on the environment**
Gary Adamkiewicz, "Buying Local: Do Food Miles Matter?" Harvard Extension School.

Page 53 *Our Farms Are at Risk*
"The Big Picture—Farming Today," The Farm Resilience Study, https://wp.wwu.edu/gigiberardi/resilient-farm-project-2009-current.

Page 54 **clover, vetch, rye, spring oats, wheat, barley**
Henning Steinfeld, Pierre Gerber, T. D. Wassenaar, Vincent Castel, Mauricio Rosales, and Cees de Haan, *Livestock's Long Shadow: Environmental Issues and Options* (Rome: Food and Agriculture Organization of the United Nations, 2006), 31, 76; and Fairlie, *Meat,* 37.

Page 54 **(as shown in Liz Carlisle's *Lentil Underground*)**
Liz Carlisle, *Lentil Underground: Renegade Farmers and the Future of Food in America* (New York: Penguin Books, 2015).

Page 54 **and biomass for the soil when decayed**

Carlisle, *Lentil Underground,* 229.

Page 55 **agrarian evangelist Joel Salatin**

Joel Salatin, *Your Successful Farm Business: Production, Profit, Pleasure* (Swoope, VA: Polyface, 2017); Joel Salatin, *The Marvelous Pigness of Pigs: Respecting and Caring for All God's Creation* (New York: Hachette Books, 2016); Joel Salatin, *Fields of Farmers: Interning, Mentoring, Partnering, Germinating* (Swoope, VA: Polyface, 2013); Joel Salatin, *Folks, This Ain't Normal: A Farmer's Advice for Happier Hens, Healthier People, and a Better World* (New York: Center Street, 2011); Joel Salatin, *The Sheer Ecstasy of Being a Lunatic Farmer* (Swoope, VA; White River Junction, VT: (Polyface, distributed by) Chelsea Green Publishing, 2010); Joel Salatin, *Everything I Want to Do Is Illegal: War Stories from the Local Food Front* (Swoope, VA: Polyface, 2007); Joel Salatin, *Holy Cows and Hog Heaven: The Food Buyer's Guide to Farm Friendly Food* (Swoope, VA; White River Junction, VT: Chelsea Green Publishing, 2005); Joel Salatin, *Family Friendly Farming: A Multigenerational Home-Based Business Testament* (Swoope, VA: Polyface, 2001); Joel Salatin, *You Can Farm: The Entrepreneur's Guide to Start & Succeed in a Farming Enterprise* (Swoope, VA: Polyface, 1998); Joel Salatin, *Pastured Poultry Profit$* (Swoope, VA: Polyface, 1996); Joel Salatin, *Salad Bar Beef* (Swoope, VA: Polyface, 1996).

Page 55 **red raspberries in 2018**

Washington Red Raspberries, "Statistics," 2018, www.red-raspberry.org/statistics.

Page 55 **Randy Honcoop**

Randy Honcoop, Structure of red raspberry production in the United States, personal communication, May 7, 2019.

Page 57 **$999,999)**

MacDonald and Hoppe, "Large Family Farms."

Page 59 **favorable fatty acid and protein composition**

Tom O'Callaghan, Deirdre Hennessy, Stephen Mcauliffe, J. Sheehan, Kieran Kilcawley, Pat Dillon, R. P. Ross, and Catherine Stanton, "The Effect of Cow Feeding System on the Composition and Quality of Milk and Dairy Products," Paper presented at the Grass-Fed Dairy Conference, Fort Plain, New York, 2018; Cynthia A. Daley, Amber Abbott, Patrick S. Doyle, Glenn A. Nader, and Stephanie Larson, "A Review of Fatty Acid Profiles and Anti-oxidant Content in Grass-Fed and Grain-Fed Beef," *Nutrition Journal* 9 (March 10, 2010): 10, https://doi.org/10.1186/1475-2891-9-10.

Page 59 ***Hard Tomatoes, Hard Times***

Jim Hightower, *Hard Tomatoes, Hard Times. A Report of the Agribusiness Accountability Project on the Failure of America's Land Grant College Complex,* Agribusiness Accountability Project (Cambridge, MA: Schenkman Publishing Co, 1973).

Page 60 has not been successful
See Barry Estabrook, *Tomatoland: How Modern Industrial Agriculture Destroyed Our Most Alluring Fruit* (Kansas City, MO: Andrews McNeel, 2011).

Page 60 reportedly millions of packages
Andrew Porterfield, "Are Seed Patent Protections Abused by Monsanto and Other Agro-Corporations?" Genetic Literacy Project, January 5, 2018.

Page 60 increases in productivity
Porterfield, "Are Seed Patent Protections Abused?"

Page 60 in India, Brazil, and elsewhere
John Seabrook, "Sowing for Apocalypse," www.newyorker.com, August 20, 2007; Vandana Shiva, ed., *Seed Sovereignty, Food Security: Women in the Vanguard of the Fight against GMOs and Corporate Agriculture* (Berkeley, CA: North Atlantic Books, 2016); Karine Peschard, "Seed Wars and Farmers' Rights: Comparative Perspectives from Brazil and India," *The Journal of Peasant Studies* 44, no. 1 (January 2, 2017): 144–68, https://doi.org/10.1080/03066150.2016.1191471; Dr. Vandana Shiva, Dr. Vinod Bhatt, Dr. Ashok Panigrahi, Kusum Mishra, Dr. Tarafdar, and Dr. Vir Singh, "Seeds of Hope, Seeds of Resilience," New Delhi, India: Navdanya/RFSTE, 2017.

Page 61 *Bread, Wine, Chocolate: The Slow Loss of Foods We Love*
Simran Sethi, *Bread, Wine, Chocolate: The Slow Loss of Foods We Love* (New York: HarperOne, 2015).

Page 61 the results are daunting
Colin K. Khoury, Anne D. Bjorkman, Hannes Dempewolf, Julian Ramirez-Villegas, Luigi Guarino, Andy Jarvis, Loren H. Rieseberg, and Paul C. Struik, "Increasing Homogeneity in Global Food Supplies and the Implications for Food Security," *Proceedings of the National Academy of Sciences* 111, no. 11 (March 18, 2014): 4001–6, https://doi.org/10.1073/pnas.1313490111.

Page 61 have evolved and changed, but its genetics have not
Fred Pearce, "The Sterile Banana," *Conservation Magazine*, September 2008; Dan Koeppel, *Banana: The Fate of the Fruit That Changed the World* (New York: Plume, 2008).

Page 61 this includes small grains and dry beans
Brook O. Brouwer, Kevin M. Murphy, and Stephen S. Jones, "Plant Breeding for Local Food Systems: A Contextual Review of End-Use Selection for Small Grains and Dry Beans in Western Washington," *Renewable Agriculture and Food Systems* 31, no. 2 (April 2016): 172–84, https://doi.org/10.1017/S1742170515000198.

Page 62 *Lentil Underground*
Carlisle, *Lentil Underground*.

Page 62 the north-central United States and southern Canada
Brouwer, Murphy, and Jones, "Plant Breeding for Local Food Systems"; Dee Goerge, "The Pulse Boom," *Successful Farming*, September 21, 2018; ckibblewhite, "Farmers

Planting More Pulse Crops Despite Market Challenges," Northern AG Network, November 16, 2018; "Vegetables & Pulses," USDA ERS, August 9, 2018.

Page 62 **"allow all eaters to buy what they want and need."**
Guthman, *Weighing In,* 195.

Page 63 **but millions more did not**
The Bureau of Agricultural Economics met an untimely end when it produced threatening research on the effects of burgeoning agribusiness—namely, a sociological survey conducted by anthropologist Walter Goldschmidt looking at the effects of farm size on the well-being of communities. The research pointed to disturbing differences in the quality of rural life as a result of increasing farm size and decreasing land tenure. These results were not welcome. There were few similar "sociological surveys" afterward, especially of a type that might be critical to agribusiness. The Farm Security Admistration eventually morphed into the more conservative Farmers' Home Administration. See Harvey M. Jacobs, ed., *Who Owns America: Social Conflict over Property Rights* (Madison: University of Wisconsin Press, 1998). Other attempts, including at one point a proposed Family Farm Development Corporation, to counter the effects of "big" and "industrial" with support for "small" have met with a similar fate—a provision to the Economic Opportunity Act of 1964 that died in committee, being replaced by a more politically acceptable emphasis on "education and training" in the War on Poverty.

Page 64 **more self-sufficiency through energy conservation**
It's worth noting that subsidies are not the only way to promote agriculture, as in the case of New Zealand. Farm subsidies were abruptly ended in New Zealand by 2009; which scale of agriculture was able to adapt most quickly, and how, is still the subject of much discussion. Some researchers found evidence of intensification and diversification (with a higher proportion of income coming from off-farm sources). Others have reported, as a result of the withholding of subsidies, less-intensive grazing of marginal land and more diversity of farm size. For more, see Berardi, Paci-Green, and Hammond, "Stability, Sustainability, and Catastrophe."

Page 65 **"Historical Overfishing and the Recent Collapse of Coastal Ecosystems,"**
Jeremy B. C. Jackson, Michael X. Kirby, Wolfgang H. Berger, Karen A. Bjorndal, Louis W. Botsford, Bruce J. Bourque, Roger H. Bradbury, et al., "Historical Overfishing and the Recent Collapse of Coastal Ecosystems," *Science* 293, no. 5530 (July 27, 2001): 629–37, https://doi.org/10.1126/science.1059199.

Page 65 **17% of the world's protein intake**
Food and Agriculture Organization of the United Nations (FAO), *The State of World Fisheries and Aquaculture: Meeting the Sustainable Development Goals,* The State of World Fisheries and Aquaculture 2018 (Rome, 2018). Also see Edward H. Allison, Allison L. Perry, Marie-Caroline Badjeck, W. Neil Adger, Katrina Brown, Declan Conway, Ashley S. Halls, et al., "Vulnerability of National Economies to the Impacts of

Climate Change on Fisheries," *Fish and Fisheries* 10, no. 2 (2009): 173–96, https://doi.org/10.1111/j.1467-2979.2008.00310.x.

Page 66 "Tragedy of the Commons" in a 1968 essay
Garrett Hardin, "The Tragedy of the Commons," *Science* 162, no. 3859 (1968): 1243–48.

Page 66 multinational management efforts have been developed
In North America, the United States collaborates with Canada to manage wide-ranging fish stocks on the west coast through agreements like the Pacific Salmon Treaty, the Pacific Fisheries Management Council, the International Pacific Halibut Commission, the Western and Central Pacific Fisheries Commission (for albacore tuna and other highly migratory species), and the Inter-American Tropical Tuna Commission. Along the Atlantic and Gulf of Mexico coasts of the United States, five other fisheries management councils coordinate regional management, including collaborating as needed with adjacent nations—Canada, Mexico, and Caribbean countries.

Page 66 in the Indian Ocean
John Vidal, "Off Tanzania, in One of the World's Richest Seas, Why Is the Catch Getting Smaller?" *The Guardian*, September 15, 2018.

Page 66 in the eastern Atlantic
Alfonso Daniels, "'Fish Are Vanishing'—Senegal's Devastated Coastline," *BBC News*, November 1, 2018.

Page 66 authorities in neighboring Mauritania
Matthew Green, "Ocean Shock: Fishmeal Factories Plunder Africa," Reuters, October 30, 2018.

Page 68 early stages of development
Lauren Kramer, "Land-Based Salmon Aquaculture: A Future with Potential," Seafood Source, October 14, 2015.

Page 69 by the USDA definition
"Food Security in the U.S.," USDA ERS, September 5, 2018.

Page 69 (the most recent data available at the time of this writing)
Alisha Coleman-Jensen, Matthew P. Rabbitt, Christian A. Gregory, and Anita Singh, "Household Food Security in the United States in 2017," USDA ERS, September 2018.

Page 70 every month in 2017 afford a nutritionally adequate diet
Center on Budget and Policy Priorities, "Policy Basics: The Supplemental Nutrition Assistance Program (SNAP)," February 13, 2018.

Page 71 relying on federal aid programs
So, for example, in my own state, Washington, in 2013, 1.3 million individuals—equivalent to a fifth of the state's population—made 8.5 million visits to food banks and pantries. On average, each client visited a food pantry 6.5 times in 2013 (Paci-Green and Berardi, "Do Global Food Systems Have an Achilles Heel?"). These statistics could be

considered an underrepresentation of the overall problem, since they do not include use of USDA's Supplemental Nutrition Assistance Program, commonly referred to as food stamps. Still, one in six households—that's 14.3%—was food insecure during 2011–2013. See Coleman-Jensen et al., "Household Food Security."

Page 71 **distribute it to over 126,000 families**
Rebekah Paci-Green and Jason Cornell, "Regional Market Research of Food Security and Regional Resilience: Whole Community Preparedness through Local Food Production and Distribution in Washington State," *Environmental Studies Faculty and Staff Publications*, 2014, 29.

Page 71 **in step with increasing food needs**
Tracie McMillan, "The New Face of Hunger," *National Geographic* (August 2014).

Page 71 **to go toward feeding the hungry**
"Food Today. Food Security Tomorrow," Feeding America, 2019.

Page 71 **$165 billion in lost dollar value**
Brad Plumer, "How the U.S. Manages to Waste $165 Billion in Food Each Year," *Washington Post*, August 22, 2012.

Page 72 **is something to work on**
For all the information here, see this excellent article: Alexandra Evans and Robin Nagele, "A Lot to Digest: Advancing Food Waste Policy in the United States," *Natural Resources Journal* 58, no. 1 (2018): 177–214. See also US EPA's "Reducing Wasted Food at Home," Overviews and Factsheets; US EPA's "United States 2030 Food Loss and Waste Reduction Goal," Overviews and Factsheets, Sustainable Management of Food; World Food Program USA, "8 Facts to Know about Food Waste and Hunger"; See also the USDA's Food Loss and Waste reduction page/site, Food and Nutrition, USDA; Adam Chandler, "Why Americans Lead the World in Food Waste," *The Atlantic*, July 15, 2016; Zach Conrad, Meredith T. Niles, Deborah A. Neher, Eric D. Roy, Nicole E. Tichenor, and Lisa Jahns, "Relationship between Food Waste, Diet Quality, and Environmental Sustainability," *PLOS ONE* 13, no. 4 (April 18, 2018): e0195405, https://doi.org/10.1371/journal.pone.0195405.

Page 72 **food deserts are everywhere**
"Go to the Atlas," USDA ERS, May 28, 2017.

Page 72 **along with race, geography, faith, and economics."**
Karen Washington, "Food Apartheid," *The Guardian*, May 15, 2018.

Page 73 **Garden-Share networks**
Amy Kepferle, "Market Share: Battling a Food Desert," *Cascadia Weekly*, July 25, 2018.

Page 73 **in his childhood neighborhood**
Michael Jackman, "Food Fighters," *Detroit Metro Times*, May 27, 2009.

Page 73 **away in the county**
Brother Nature Produce, 2019, http://brothernatureproduce.com/about.html.

Page 74 **big cities and rural areas**

"Key Statistics & Graphics," Food Security in the U.S. See also Constance Gordon and Kathleen Hunt, "Reform, Justice, and Sovereignty: A Food Systems Agenda for Environmental Communication," *Environmental Communication* 13, no. 1 (January 2, 2019): 9–22, https://doi.org/10.1080/17524032.2018.1435559.

Page 74 **who is most vulnerable**

See also: Grace Tatter, "Food Insecurity on College Campuses," Harvard Graduate School of Education, November 15, 2018.

Page 74 **not going to reduce food insecurity**

Rachel Louise Moran, "Why American Policy Is Leaving Millions Hungry," *Washington Post*, August 7, 2018; Craig Gundersen and James P. Ziliak, "Food Insecurity Research in the United States: Where We Have Been and Where We Need to Go," *Applied Economic Perspectives and Policy* 40, no. 1 (March 1, 2018): 119–35, https://doi .org/10.1093/aepp/ppx058.

Page 74 **$70 billion on food assistance programs**

Center on Budget and Policy Priorities, Policy Basics.

PART 2

Page 79 **omega-3 fatty acids**

National Institutes of Health Office of Dietary Supplements, "Omega-3 Fatty Acids: Fact Sheet for Health Professionals," last updated July 9, 2019.

Page 82 **hefty antioxidant load**

Elisa Tripoli, Marco Giammanco, Garden Tabacchi, Danila Di Majo, Santo Giammanco, and Maurizio La Guardia, "The Phenolic Compounds of Olive Oil: Structure, Biological Activity and Beneficial Effects on Human Health," *Nutrition Research Reviews* 18, no. 1 (June 2005): 98–112, https://doi.org/10.1079/NRR200495.

Page 83 **affects how much food you consume?**

See, for example, Patricia O. Williamson, Larry Lockshin, I. Leigh Francis, and Simone Mueller Loose, "Influencing Consumer Choice: Short and Medium Term Effect of Country of Origin Information on Wine Choice," *Food Quality and Preference* 51 (July 1, 2016): 89–99, https://doi.org/10.1016/j.foodqual.2016.02.018.

Page 83 **we frequent and how often**

It is difficult to measure media exposure, but this article makes an attempt to assess methods: Claes H. de Vreese and Peter Neijens, "Measuring Media Exposure in a Changing Communications Environment," *Communication Methods and Measures* 10, no. 2–3 (April 2, 2016): 69–80, https://doi.org/10.1080/19312458.2016.1150441.

Page 83 **particularly susceptible to advertising**
Frans Folkvord, Doeschka J. Anschütz, Reinout W. Wiers, and Moniek Buijzen, "The Role of Attentional Bias in the Effect of Food Advertising on Actual Food Intake among Children," *Appetite* 84 (January 1, 2015): 251–58, https://doi.org/10.1016/j.appet.2014.10.016.

Page 84 **drinking more cups per day**
Simran Sethi, "A Surprising New Trend in Coffee," *Forbes*, December 1, 2017.

Page 84 **part of Starbucks's messaging, too**
Christine Champagne and Teressa Iezzi, "Dunkin Donuts and Starbucks: A Tale of Two Coffee Marketing Giants," *Fast Company*, August 21, 2014; see, for fair trade issues, Barbara Kessler, GreenRightNow, "A Starbucks Boycott Percolates over Fair Trade and Organic Ingredients," Binghamton Homepage, July 23, 2015.

Page 84 **over 42 gallons per person**
Beverage Marketing Corporation, "Consumers Reaffirm Bottled Water Is America's Favorite Drink," *The BMC Beverage Blog*, May 31, 2018.

Page 86 **Sandor Katz**
Sandor Ellix Katz, *The Revolution Will Not Be Microwaved: Inside America's Underground Food Movements*, 1st edition (White River Junction, VT: Chelsea Green Publishing, 2006); Sandor Ellix Katz, *The Art of Fermentation: An In-Depth Exploration of Essential Concepts and Processes from around the World* (White River Junction, VT: Chelsea Green Publishing, 2012).

Page 86 **purchases that required preparation."**
Federation of American Societies for Experimental Biology, "Highly processed foods dominate U.S. grocery purchases," *ScienceDaily*, March 29, 2015.

Page 87 *Twinkie, Deconstructed* author Steve Ettlinger
Ettlinger, *Twinkie, Deconstructed*.

Page 87 **chemical leavening and faster baking**
For some demographics, convenience can literally make the difference between food and hunger. The book by Julie A. Caswell and Ann L. Yaktine, *Supplemental Nutrition Assistance Program: Examining the Evidence to Define Benefit Adequacy* (Washington, DC: National Academies Press, 2013), gives detailed information on the adequacy of nutrition provided for those in income transfer programs, and mentions prepared foods.

Page 87 **cruise down those convenience store aisles**
Other important works followed: Marion Nestle, *Food Politics: How the Food Industry Influences Nutrition and Health* (Berkeley, CA: University of California Press, 2002); see also Marion Nestle, *What to Eat* (New York: North Point Press, 2006); *Safe Food: The Politics of Food Safety* (Berkeley, CA: University of California Press, 2003); *Why Calories Count: From Science to Politics* (Berkeley, CA: University of California Press, 2012); *Unsavory Truth: How Food Companies Skew the Science of What We Eat* (New York: Hachette Book Group,

2018); *Eat, Drink, Vote: An Illustrated Guide to Food Politics* (New York: Rodale, 2013); and *Soda Politics: Taking on Big Soda (and Winning)* (New York: Oxford University Press, 2015).

Page 87 **7,000 items in a grocery store to more like 40–50,000**
Michael Ruhlman, *The Buying and Selling of Food in America* (New York: Abrams, 2017).

Page 87 *Salt Sugar Fat: How the Food Giants Hooked Us*
Michael Moss, *Salt Sugar Fat: How the Food Giants Hooked Us,* Reprint edition (New York: Random House Trade Paperbacks, 2014).

Page 89 **Ghastly the mouth and gums enormous swell'd…**
From the *Lusiad* by Luís de Camões, writing about Vasco da Gama's expedition. See Jason Mayberry, "Scurvy and Vitamin C" (Harvard Library, 2004).

Page 89 **as early as the 1400s**
Gavin Menzies, *1421: The Year China Discovered America* (New York: William Morrow Paperbacks, 2008).

Page 89 **better intake of protein**
Kenneth F. Kiple and Kriemhild Conee Ornelas, eds., *The Cambridge World History of Food* (Cambridge: Cambridge University Press, 2008), https://doi.org/10.1017/CHOL9780521402149.

Page 90 *In Defense of Food*
Pollan, *In Defense of Food.*

Page 90 **nutritionism, using a USDA Handbook**
USDA Handbook, 1976–1992; "Index to USDA Agriculture Handbooks," USDA, May 1992.

Page 91 **the sum of all the food you eat**
Dieting is in our cultural genetics. For well over 2,000 years, people have dieted to promote mental and physical health. The ancient Greek *diaita* was a lifestyle concept of food, exercise, and leisure.

Page 91 **$60-billion diet industry**
Linda Searing, "The Big Number: 45 Million Americans Go on a Diet Each Year," *Washington Post,* January 1, 2018. The number $60 billion was also given in Adela Hruby and Frank B. Hu, "The Epidemiology of Obesity: A Big Picture," *PharmacoEconomics* 33, no. 7 (July 2015): 673–89, https://doi.org/10.1007/s40273-014-0243-x.

Page 92 **with sometimes disastrous effects**
Daniel Eisenberg, Emily J. Nicklett, Kathryn Roeder, and Nina E. Kirz, "Eating Disorder Symptoms Among College Students: Prevalence, Persistence, Correlates, and Treatment-Seeking," *Journal of American College Health* 59, no. 8 (November 2011): 700–707, https://doi.org/10.1080/07448481.2010.546461.

Page 92 **important contributors**
Michael P. Levine and Linda Smolak, "Prevention of Negative Body Image, Disordered Eating, and Eating Disorders: An Update," in *Annual Review of Eating Disorders: Pt. 1,*

eds. Stephen Wonderlich, James Mitchell, and Martine de Zwaan (London: CRC Press, 2007), 1-13; see also Mia L. Pellizzer, Marika Tiggemann, Glenn Waller, and Tracey D. Wade, "Measures of Body Image: Confirmatory Factor Analysis and Association with Disordered Eating." *Psychological Assessment* 30, no. 2 (February 2018): 143–53, https://doi.org/10.1037/pas0000461.

Page 92 *Weighing In: Obesity, Food Justice, and the Limits of Capitalism*
Guthman, *Weighing In.*

Page 93 **show what was expected**
"Low-Fat Diet Not a Cure-All," T. H. Chan School of Public Health, February 9, 2006.

Page 93 **did not appear to reduce these**
Cheryl Ritenbaugh, Ruth E. Patterson, Rowan T. Chlebowski, Bette Caan, Lesley Fels-Tinker, Barbara Howard, and Judy Ockene, "The Women's Health Initiative Dietary Modification Trial: Overview and Baseline Characteristics of Participants," *Annals of Epidemiology* 13, no. 9 (October 2003): S87–97, https://doi.org/10.1016/S1047-2797(03)00044-9.

Page 93 **this poor attempt to restrict calories**
Some material in this paragraph is from Berardi, *Finding Balance.*

Page 94 **making serious lifestyle as well as food changes**
"The National Weight Control Registry," www.nwcr.ws.

Page 95 **as Daniel Patrick Moynihan memorably put it**
Daniel Patrick Moynihan, "An American Original," *The Hive,* www.vanityfair.com.

Page 95 **and paraded as scientific reporting**
Rheana Murray, "Egg Yolks Almost as Bad for Your Heart as Smoking Cigarettes, Says Study," *New York Daily News,* August 17, 2012.

Page 96 **include them in diets**
Mitchell M. Kanter, Penny M. Kris-Etherton, Maria Luz Fernandez, Kasey C. Vickers, and David L. Katz, "Exploring the Factors That Affect Blood Cholesterol and Heart Disease Risk: Is Dietary Cholesterol as Bad for You as History Leads Us to Believe?" *Advances in Nutrition* 3, no. 5 (September 1, 2012): 711–17, https://doi.org/10.3945/an.111.001321.

Page 96 **cast doubt on the effects of eggs**
For example, studies that found "no adverse association between dietary cholesterol and serum lipid levels or cardiovascular risk amongst those with impaired fasting glucose or Type 2 diabetes." Yinhong Chen and Ronald R. Watson, "Effect of Dietary Eggs on Human Serum Cholesterol and Coronary Heart Disease," in *Eggs and Health Promotion* ed. Ronald R. Watson (Ames, IA: Iowa State Press, 2002), 101-109.

Page 97 blamed fat as a health hazard
Cristin E. Kearns, Laura A. Schmidt, and Stanton A. Glantz, "Sugar Industry and Coronary Heart Disease Research," *JAMA Internal Medicine* 126, no. 11 (2016): 1680–85.

Page 97 of the research itself
See: Lenard Lesser, Cara B. Ebbeling, Merrill Goozner, David Wypij, and David Ludwig, "Relationship between Funding Source and Conclusion among Nutrition-Related Scientific Articles," *PLoS Medicine* 4 (February 1, 2007): e5, https://doi.org/10.1371/journal.pmed.0040005.

Page 98 lean meats, fruits and vegetables, and olive oil
See Jane E. Brody, "Dr. Ancel Keys, 100, Promoter of Mediterranean Diet, Dies," *New York Times*, November 23, 2004.

Page 98 *Eat Well and Stay Well*
Ancel Keys and Margaret Keys, *Eat Well and Stay Well* (New York: Doubleday, 1959).

Page 99 *Obesity, and Disease*
Robert Lustig, *Fat Chance: Beating the Odds against Sugar, Processed Food, Obesity, and Disease* (New York: Penguin Books, 2013).

Page 99 person's serum cholesterol."
William P. Castelli, "Concerning the Possibility of a Nut...," *Archives of Internal Medicine* 152, no. 7 (July 1, 1992): 1371, https://doi.org/10.1001/archinte.1992.00400190013003.

Page 99 continue to offer new insights
See Connie W. Tsao and Ramachandran S. Vasan, "The Framingham Heart Study: Past, Present and Future," *International Journal of Epidemiology* 44, no. 6 (2015): 1763–66.

Page 100 provocative results to stir you to dig deeper
For a very instructive essay on how the science world works, with a cast of characters including people mentioned here, see Ian Leslie, "The Sugar Conspiracy," *The Guardian*, April 7, 2016.

Page 102 *The Omnivore's Dilemma*
Michael Pollan, *The Omnivore's Dilemma* (New York: Penguin Press, 2006).

Page 102 20:1 of our contemporary grain-fed beef-based diets
A. P. Simopoulos, "Evolutionary Aspects of Diet, the Omega-6/Omega-3 Ratio and Genetic Variation: Nutritional Implications for Chronic Diseases," *Biomedicine & Pharmacotherapy* 60, no. 9 (November 2006): 502–7, https://doi.org/10.1016/j.biopha.2006.07.080. Also see Cynthia A. Daley, Amber Abbott, Patrick S. Doyle, Glenn A. Nader, and Stephanie Larson, "A Review of Fatty Acid Profiles and Antioxidant Content in Grass-Fed and Grain-Fed Beef," *Nutrition Journal* 9 (March 10, 2010): 10, https://doi.org/10.1186/1475-2891-9-10.

Page 102 hydrogenation process
For example, hydrogenation (adding hydrogen to a fat in a chemically controlled process, with the aid of a catalyst) increases the overall hardness of the processed food—think margarine from vegetable oils.

Page 102 **for butter, lard, and tallow**

Trans fats are currently being monitored (labeling helps) and are being phased out. See Rebecca Voelker, "Partially Hydrogenated Oils Are Out," *JAMA* 314, no. 5 (August 4, 2015): 443, https://doi.org/10.1001/jama.2015.8387. Also see these excellent works: Amy C. Brown, *Understanding Food: Principles and Preparation,* 6th edition (Boston: Cengage, 2019); K. Warner, "Impact of High-Temperature Food Processing on Fats and Oils," *Advances in Experimental Medicine and Biology* 459 (1999): 67–77; and Jeya Henry, "Processing, Manufacturing, Uses and Labelling of Fats in the Food Supply," *Annals of Nutrition and Metabolism* 55, no. 1–3 (2009): 273–300, https://doi.org/10.1159/000229006. It was Harvard University's Walter Willet and colleagues, and before that, Mary Enig and colleagues, who identified negative nutritional effects of trans fats in processed foods. See M. G. Enig, S. Atal, M. Keeney, and J. Sampugna, "Isomeric Trans Fatty Acids in the U.S. Diet," *Journal of the American College of Nutrition* 9, no. 5 (October 1990): 471–86, https://doi.org/10.1080/07315724.1990.10720404; W. C. Willett, M. J. Stampfer, J. E. Manson, G. A. Colditz, F. E. Speizer, B. A. Rosner, L. A. Sampson, and C. H. Hennekens, "Intake of Trans Fatty Acids and Risk of Coronary Heart Disease among Women," *The Lancet* 341, no. 8845 (March 6, 1993): 581–85.

Page 103 **we have too much of**

In fact, artificial trans fats in food have been banned by the FDA since June 2018. However, foods manufactured prior to the ban can be distributed for another couple of years, and foods with less than 0.5 grams of trans fats per serving still can be labeled as having 0 grams of trans fats. See an early report on the ban: Sabrina Tavernise, "F.D.A. Sets 2018 Deadline to Rid Foods of Trans Fats," *New York Times,* December 21, 2017; and more recent popular articles in Daisy Coyle, "7 Foods That Still Contain Trans Fats," *Healthline Newsletter,* October 29, 2018 and Kathleen Doheny, "FDA: Farewell to Trans Fats," WebMD, accessed May 8, 2019.

Page 104 **both cholesterol sulfate and vitamin D) makes things worse**

Stephanie Seneff, Glyn Wainwright, and Luca Mascitelli, "Is the Metabolic Syndrome Caused by a High Fructose, and Relatively Low-fat, Low Cholesterol Diet?" *Archives of Medical Science* 7, no. 1 (2011): 8–20; Robert M. Davidson and Stephanie Seneff, "The Initial Common Pathway of Inflammation, Disease, and Sudden Death," *Entropy* 14 (2012): 1399–442; Stephanie Seneff, Ann Lauritzen, Robert Davidson, and Laurie Lentz-Marino, "Is Endothelial Nitric Oxide Synthase a Moonlighting Protein Whose Day Job Is Cholesterol Sulfate Synthesis? Implications for Cholesterol Transport, Diabetes and Cardiovascular Disease," *Entropy* 14, no. 12 (December 2012): 2492–530, https://doi.org/10.3390/e14122492; Stephanie Seneff, Robert M. Davidson, and Jingjing Liu, "Is Cholesterol Sulfate Deficiency a Common Factor in Preeclampsia, Autism, and Pernicious Anemia?" *Entropy* 14, (2012): 2265–90; and Stephanie Seneff, Robert M. Davidson, Ann Lauritzen, Anthony Samsel, and Glyn Wainwright, "A Novel Hypothesis for Atherosclerosis as a Cholesterol Sulfate Deficiency Syndrome,"

Theoretical Biology & Medical Modelling 12 (May 27, 2015): 9, https://doi.org/10.1186/s12976-015-0006-1.

Page 105 **nerve fibers**
"Effects of Starvation on the Central Nervous System," *Nutrition Reviews* 9, no. 7 (July 1, 1951): 202–4, https://doi.org/10.1111/j.1753-4887.1951.tb02632.x.

Page 105 **an endocrine organ itself**
Hitoshi Nishizawa and Iichiro Shimomura, "Fat Cell Lipolysis and Future Weight Gain," *Journal of Diabetes Investigation* 10, no. 2 (March 2019): 221–23, https://doi.org/10.1111/jdi.12950; J. Michael Gonzalez-Campoy, Daniel L. Hurley, and W. Timothy Garvey, eds., *Bariatric Endocrinology: Evaluation and Management of Adiposity, Adiposopathy and Related Diseases* (New York: Springer, 2018).

Page 106 **whole and refined grains)**
Some of this information is in Berardi, *Finding Balance*. Dancers were the first population for which I wrote on diet, health, and nutrition. Since then, much on these topics has been written for dancers, arguably, one of the most vulnerable populations at risk for disordered eating. See a more recent text on the subject: Liane Simmel and Eva-Maria Kraft, *Nutrition for Dancers: Basics, Performance Enhancement, Practical Tips* (New York: Routledge, 2017).

Page 107 **20% sweeter than white table sugar**
Sam Z. Sun, G. Harvey Anderson, Brent D. Flickinger, Patricia S. Williamson-Hughes, and Mark W. Empie, "Fructose and Non-Fructose Sugar Intakes in the US Population and Their Associations with Indicators of Metabolic Syndrome," *Food and Chemical Toxicology* 49, no. 11 (November 2011): 2875–82, https://doi.org/10.1016/j.fct.2011.07.068.

Page 107 **our health problems**
See University of California San Francisco, "How Much Is Too Much?" Sugarscience: the unsweetened truth (website), https://sugarscience.ucsf.edu; New Hampshire Department of Health and Human Service, "How Much Sugar Do You Eat? You May Be Surprised!" (NH DHHS-DPHS-Health Promotion in Motion).

Page 107 **our current consumption**
A good source for authoritative reviews of the science on sugar is the website, Sugarscience: the unsweetened truth, https://sugarscience.ucsf.edu, from the University of California, San Francisco.

Page 107 **a can of soda."**
Robert Lustig, "Sweet Revenge," https://robertlustig.com/sweet-revenge.

Page 107 **we want more and more**
See Robert H. Lustig's discussion in his book, *The Hacking of the American Mind: The Science Behind the Corporate Takeover of Our Bodies and Brains* (New York: Penguin Books, 2017). Note the idea of sugar as addictive is somewhat contested; see Margaret L.

Westwater, Paul C. Fletcher, and Hisham Ziauddeen, "Sugar Addiction: The State of the Science," *European Journal of Nutrition* 55, no. Suppl 2 (November 2016): 55–69, https://doi.org/10.1007/s00394-016-1229-6.

Page 107 **"Sugar: The Bitter Truth"**
Robert Lustig, "Sugar: The Bitter Truth," University of California TV, 2009.

Page 107 *Fat Chance*
Lustig, *Fat Chance.*

Page 108 **since ghrelin levels stay high**
Kathleen A. Page, Owen Chan, Jagriti Arora, Renata Belfort-Deaguiar, James Dzuira, Brian Roehmholdt, Gary W. Cline, et al., "Effects of Fructose vs Glucose on Regional Cerebral Blood Flow in Brain Regions Involved with Appetite and Reward Pathways," *JAMA* 309, no. 1 (January 2, 2013): 63–70, https://doi.org/10.1001/jama.2012.116975.

Page 108 *The Hacking of the American Mind: The Science Behind the Corporate Takeover of Our Bodies and Brains*
Lustig, *The Hacking of the American Mind.*

Page 109 **and you'll be happy**
Lustig has his "fructose-believer" critics, as some don't appreciate his finger-pointing at fructose and its "dangers." See, for example: Tauseef A. Khan and John L. Sievenpiper, "Controversies about Sugars: Results from Systematic Reviews and Meta-Analyses on Obesity, Cardiometabolic Disease and Diabetes," *European Journal of Nutrition* 55, no. Suppl 2 (November 2016): 25–43, https://doi.org/10.1007/s00394-016-1345-3. These critics are perhaps more gracious than blog/social media pundits, some also biting in their criticism.

Page 109 **that ropes in so many of us**
There's an interesting discussion of many of these issues here: Gary Taubes, "Is Sugar Toxic?" *New York Times,* April 13, 2011.

Page 110 **from time to time**
See Anahad O'Connor, "How the Sugar Industry Shifted Blame to Fat," *New York Times,* December 21, 2017. Importantly, Marion Nestle thoughtfully critiqued industry funding of research in an editorial at the time the paper revealing the sugar industry/Harvard links was published. See Marion Nestle, "Food Industry Funding of Nutrition Research: The Relevance of History for Current Debates," *JAMA Internal Medicine* 176, no. 11 (November 1, 2016): 1685–86, https://doi.org/10.1001/jamainternmed.2016.5400.

Page 111 **in World War II**
See Jacob Lahne, "Sensory Science, the Food Industry, and the Objectification of Taste," *Anthropology of Food,* no. 10 (January 28, 2016). Lahne is on the faculty at Virginia Tech, College of Agriculture and Life Sciences.

Page 113 of food affects consumer responses

A much larger study that Erminio Monteleone and Caterina Dinnella are working on now is "Italian Taste"—a multi-year large-scale project coordinated by the Italian Sensory Science Society, of which Monteleone is president, involving eighteen labs, and aimed at exploring individual differences in food preference and food-related behavior among Italians. See the project website, www.it-taste.it, especially publications.

Pages 113–114 what is actually offered to the consumer."

Claudio Peri, "Quality Excellence in Extra Virgin Olive Oils," in *Olive Oil Sensory Science*, eds. Erminio Monteleone and Susan Langstaff (John Wiley & Sons, Ltd, 2013), 4, https://doi.org/10.1002/9781118332511.ch1.

Page 114 presence of certain chemicals like free fatty acids

"United States Standards for Grades of Olive Oil and Olive-Pomace Oil," USDA, October 25, 2010.

Page 115 Carlo Petrini did

Petrini, *Slow Food Nation*.

PART 3

Page 121 artificial trans fats

See Mayo Clinic Staff, "Trans Fat: Double Trouble for Your Heart," Mayo Clinic, www.mayoclinic.org.

Page 121 on grass

University of California Berkeley Wellness, "Grass-Fed Beef for Omega-3s?" January 7, 2015.

Page 122 "nobody needs, but everyone craves."

Alexander Bentley, Mark Horton, and Philip Langton, "A History of Sugar—the Food Nobody Needs, but Everyone Craves," The Conversation, October 30, 2015.

Page 122 sugar consumed by Americans

Or 39%, to be precise. See U.S. Department of Health and Human Services and U.S. Department of Agriculture, 2015–2020 Dietary Guidelines for Americans, 8th edition, December 2015.

Page 122 especially sugary drinks—that's a problem

Information on this topic, besides Lustig's work, is readily available: Jeffrey B. Schwimmer, Patricia Ugalde-Nicalo, Jean A. Welsh, Jorge E. Angeles, Maria Cordero, Kathryn E. Harlow, Adina Alazraki, et al., "Effect of a Low Free Sugar Diet vs Usual Diet on Non-alcoholic Fatty Liver Disease in Adolescent Boys: A Randomized Clinical Trial," *JAMA* 321, no. 3 (January 22, 2019): 256–65, https://doi.org/10.1001/jama.2018.20579; and discussed fairly well here: Anahad O'Connor, "To Fight Fatty Liver, Avoid Sugary Foods and Drinks," *New York Times*, January 29, 2019.

Page 122 **spike of dopamine it delivers**
Javier Franco-Pérez, Joaquín Manjarrez-Marmolejo, Paola Ballesteros-Zebadúa, Adriana Neri-Santos, Sergio Montes, Norma Suarez-Rivera, Miguel Hernández-Cerón, and Vadim Pérez-Koldenkova, "Chronic Consumption of Fructose Induces Behavioral Alterations by Increasing Orexin and Dopamine Levels in the Rat Brain," *Nutrients* 10, no. 11 (November 10, 2018), https://doi.org/10.3390/nu10111722.

Page 124 **throughout the entire agricultural web**
Michaël Wilde, "True Cost Accounting Pilot Calculates Hidden Impacts of Food on People and Planet," eosta: where ecology meets economy, June 13, 2017; European Commission and Directorate-General for Health and Consumer Protection, *Food Traceability*, 2007.

Page 127 **as much as by plane**
Berners-Lee, *How Bad Are Bananas?*

Page 127 **price advantage**
Adamkiewicz, "Buying Local."

Page 127 **most of which are grown by large-scale farms**
See the price support critique in the *Star Tribune:* Andy Brehm, "Opinion Exchange: Sugar Subsidies Are Sweet, but Not for the Taxpayer," *Star Tribune,* October 6, 2013.

Page 129 **vats affect the quality of each cheese**
Giuseppe Licitra, Margherita Caccamo, Florence Valence, and Sylvie Lortal, "Traditional Wooden Equipment Used for Cheesemaking and Their Effect on Quality," in *Global Cheesemaking Technology,* eds. Photis Papademas and Thomas Bintsis (Chichester, UK: John Wiley & Sons, Ltd, 2017), 157–72, https://doi.org/10.1002/9781119046165.ch0g.

Page 130 **author of** *Diet for a Small Planet*
Frances Moore Lappé, *Diet for a Small Planet* (New York: Ballantine, 1971).

Page 131 *How to Cook a Wolf*
Fisher, *How to Cook a Wolf.*

Page 131 *An Everlasting Meal: Cooking with Economy and Grace*
Tamar Adler, *An Everlasting Meal: Cooking with Economy and Grace* (New York: Scribner, 2011).

Page 132 **involve the most harmful growing practices**
Environmental Working Group, "Shopper's Guide."

Page 132 **deforestation and pesticide poisonings**
See this article and the comments that follow it: AFP, "Mexico's Avocado Boom Causing Deforestation and Illnesses in Local Population, Experts Say," *The Independent,* November 4, 2016.

Page 139 **pesticide-contaminated produce**
Environmental Working Group, "Shopper's Guide."

Page 141 **the lack of pesticides is a big deal**

Damian Carrington, "Buy Organic Food to Help Curb Global Insect Collapse, Say Scientists," *The Guardian,* February 13, 2019.

Page 142 **organically bred seeds**

Johannes Wirz, Peter Kunz, and Ueli Hurter, "Seed as a Commons, Breeding as a Source for Real Economy, Law and Culture" (Goetheanum and Fund for Crop Development, 2017).

Page 142 **to make it happen**

Viva Farms, "Farm Business Incubator," https://vivafarms.org/farm-business-incubator.

Page 143 **better decisions about food**

See Barry Schwartz and Kenneth Sharpe, *Practical Wisdom: The Right Way to Do the Right Thing* (New York: Riverhead Books, 2011). For *FoodWISE,* I have drawn heavily on *Practical Wisdom* and other writings of Barry Schwartz and Kenneth Sharpe on the general topic of experience and practical wisdom, and the strong relationship between the two. In a discussion with Barry Schwartz at Swarthmore College during the 2013–2014 academic year, I asked him if he had thought about applying the idea of experience, and "practical food wisdom," to his work on institutions failing to do the right thing (usually by focusing on rules and regulations rather than experience and wise judgment). "Only at the dinner table," he replied—which got me thinking that I could and should apply such thinking to what could best be called a FoodWISE approach.

PART 4

Page 147 **largest carbon footprint either)**

Adamkiewicz, "Buying Local."

Page 153 *New Yorker's* **"Raw Faith" article**

Burkhard Bilger, "Raw Faith," *New Yorker,* August 19, 2002.

Page 153 **Harvard public lecture series**

"Sister Noella Marcellino, "Tales from the Cheese Caves" (Harvard University Science & Cooking Public Lecture Series, 2016), www.youtube.com/watch?v=1sdBFqIsX1Q. Here, as in her published work, Noella Marcellino and David R. Benson, "The Good, the Bad, and the Ugly: Tales of Mold-Ripened Cheese," in *Cheese and Microbes,* ed. Catherine W. Donnelly (American Society for Microbiology, 2014), 95–131, Sister Noella presents her research on the ecology (and great diversity) of natural cheese-ripening microbes in traditional cheese-ripening caves. The diversity of the fungi whose enzymes impact cheese aroma and texture likely contribute to the great variety of French cheeses. Sister Noella encourages American artisanal cheesemakers to take advantage of and increase—by managing temperature, humidity, and other factors of aging—the biodiversity present in their cheese-ripening environments. For references on her early work, highlighting the diversity of *Geotrichum candidum* as a cheese-ripening fungus, see N. Marcellino, E. Beuvier, R. Grappin, M. Guéguen, and D. R. Benson. "Diversity of *Geotrichum Candidum* Strains Isolated from Traditional Cheesemaking Fabrications in France." *Applied and Environmental Microbiology* 67, no. 10 (October 1, 2001): 4752–59, https://doi.org/10.1128/AEM.67.10.4752-4759.2001.

Page 153 Michael Pollan's book *Cooked*
Michael Pollan, *Cooked: A Natural History of Transformation* (New York: Penguin Books, 2013).

Page 154 *Joy of Cooking*
Irma S. Rombauer, Marion Rombauer Becker, and Ethan Becker, *Joy of Cooking,* 75th anniversary edition (New York: Scribner, 2006).

Page 154 *Nourishing Traditions)*
Sally Fallon and Mary G. Enig, *Nourishing Traditions: The Cookbook That Challenges Politically Correct Nutrition and Diet Dictocrats,* 2nd edition (Washington, DC: Newtrends Publishing, Inc., 2001).

Page 155 high-grade raw milk in my home state of Washington
To get information on commercial availability where you live, see "Real Milk Finder," A Campaign for Real Milk: A Project of the Weston A. Price Foundation, www.realmilk.com/real-milk-finder.

Page 155 problems recovering the solids
See "Problems with Ultra Pasteurized Milk," New England Cheesemaking Supply Company, https://cheesemaking.com/blogs/fun-along-the-whey/problems-with-ultra-pasteurized-milk for a good description of what kind of solids recovery you might expect; or, see my online cheese course taught with ecotoxicologist and good colleague Ruth Sofield: "Summer Session," Western Washington University Extended Education, https://ee.wwu.edu/summer-session.

Page 157 countries like Peru and Bolivia
Jeremy Cherfas, "Your Quinoa Habit Really Did Help Peru's Poor. But There's Trouble Ahead," *NPR,* March 31, 2016.

Page 157 a hundred years ago
Donald D. Kasarda, "Can an Increase in Celiac Disease Be Attributed to an Increase in the Gluten Content of Wheat as a Consequence of Wheat Breeding?" *Journal of Agricultural and Food Chemistry* 61, no. 6 (February 13, 2013): 1155–59, https://doi.org/10.1021/jf305122s.

Page 158 made with refined flours
"Going with the Grain," Washington State University Bread Lab, http://thebreadlab.wsu.edu/going-with-the-grain.

Page 158 connected to gluten consumption
See this article: Michael Specter, "Against the Grain," *New Yorker,* October 27, 2014.

Page 158 *The Tassajara Bread Book*
Brown, *Tassajara Bread Book.*

Page 163 **Nourishing Foods advocate Sally Fallon**
Fallon and Enig, *Nourishing Traditions.*

Page 163 **industrial scale as well**
California produces about 80% of the world's commercial almond crop on about one million acres—which requires one and a half to two million beehives to pollinate, which, in turn are a good chunk, maybe two-thirds or more, of US total beehives. See: Emily Wilder, "Bees for Hire: California Almonds Become Migratory Colonies' Biggest Task," Stanford University/The Bill Lane Center for the American West, August 17, 2018; Brittney Goodrich, "A Bee Economist Explains Honey Bees' Vital Role in Growing Tasty Almonds," The Conversation, August 17, 2018; James Hamblin, "The Dark Side of Almond Use," *The Atlantic,* August 28, 2014. These bees are livestock, indirectly producing food in the form of the almonds (and, doing other incidental things like pollinating other crops and making honey later in the summer). Each almond requires over a gallon of water to grow, and California, chronically in drought, is using 44% more land for almonds than ten years ago, stressing other water users—like the endangered salmon in northern California's Klamath River (see Hamblin, *The Dark Side).* Pesticides, also used on almond trees, have to be carefully managed to avoid harming the bees.

Page 165 **Teresa Rieland of sweetveg**
Teresa Rieland, sweetveg, https://sweetveg.org.

Page 169 *Diet for a Small Planet*
Lappé, *Diet for a Small Planet.*

Page 169 **the lowest setting on a Crock-Pot)**
Kristen Michaelis, "Is Pressure Cooking Healthy?" Food Renegade, www.foodrenegade.com.

Page 172 **over 75% of total world production**
Hayley Boriss, "Commodity Profile: Garlic" (Agricultural Marketing Resource Center, January 2006), https://aic.ucdavis.edu/wp-content/uploads/2019/01/agmr-profile-Garlic-2006B.pdf.

Page 172 **hefty price in terms of social costs**
Yuan Yang, "Supply Chains: The Dirty Secret of China's Prisons," *Financial Times,* August 29, 2019.

Page 194 **adapted from a *New York Times* recipe**
Melissa Clark, "Salt-and-Pepper Roast Chicken Recipe," NYT Cooking, https://cooking.nytimes.com.

Page 201 **Teresa Rieland of sweetveg**
Teresa Rieland, sweetveg, https://sweetveg.org.

INDEX

ABOUT THE AUTHOR

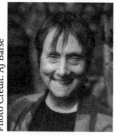

GIGI BERARDI is a professor at Western Washington University's Huxley College of the Environment and director of the Resilient Farm Project. She has taught food and geography classes in Europe, Mexico, Lummi Nation, and several universities and colleges in the United States. She homesteads in the summer in Washington's San Juan Islands, where she milks sheep and makes cheese. Berardi maintains a popular food blog (https://wp.wwu.edu /gigiberardi/category/foodwise-resilient-farms-and-nourishing-foods-blog/). She also has published in numerous scientific journals such as *BioScience, Ethnohistory, Human Ecology Review, Journal of Sustainable Agriculture*, and *Society and Natural Resources*. Her articles and reviews have appeared in newspapers (*Anchorage Daily News, Los Angeles Times, The Olympian*), and her public radio features (for KSKA, Anchorage, Alaska) have been recognized by the Society of Professional Journalists.

Berardi received her bachelor's degree in biology from the University of California San Diego and master's and doctoral degrees from Cornell University in natural resources policy and planning. She was a Fulbright scholar in Italy. She also holds a master's in dance from the University of California Los Angeles, which is the basis for her popular book, *Finding Balance*, and much of her other writing in dance. Berardi is an elected member of the American Society of Journalists and Authors.